THE 10-WEEK
INTELLIGENT
FITNESS
CHALLENGE

Also by Simon Waterson and published by
Michael O'Mara Books

Intelligent Fitness: The Smart Way
to Reboot Your Body and Get in Shape

THE 10-WEEK INTELLIGENT FITNESS CHALLENGE

The Ultimate Workout Programme from Hollywood's Most In-demand Trainer

SIMON WATERSON
with a foreword by TOM HIDDLESTON

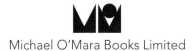

Michael O'Mara Books Limited

For B, H and O xxx
And for P, A and O xxx

First published in Great Britain in 2023
by Michael O'Mara Books Limited
9 Lion Yard
Tremadoc Road
London SW4 7NQ

A CIP catalogue record for this book is available from
the British Library.

Papers used by Michael O'Mara Books Limited are
natural, recyclable products made from wood grown
in sustainable forests. The manufacturing processes
conform to the environmental regulations of the
country of origin.

ISBN: 978-1-78929-506-1 in paperback print format
ISBN: 978-1-78929-507-8 in ebook format

2 3 4 5 6 7 8 9 10

www.mombooks.com

Designed and typeset by Ana Bjezancevic

Front cover and workout photography by
Eddy Massarella
Photographs of Tom Hiddleston and photograph of
Simon on this page © Greg Williams

Printed and bound by Bell & Bain Ltd, Glasgow, UK

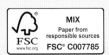

MIX
Paper from
responsible sources
FSC® C007785
FSC
www.fsc.org

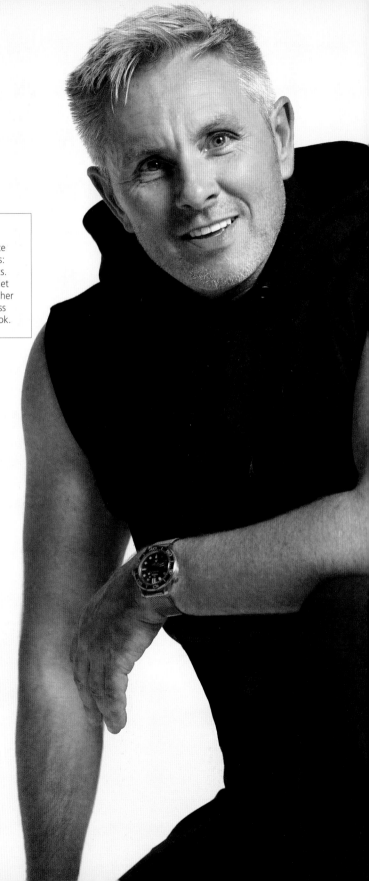

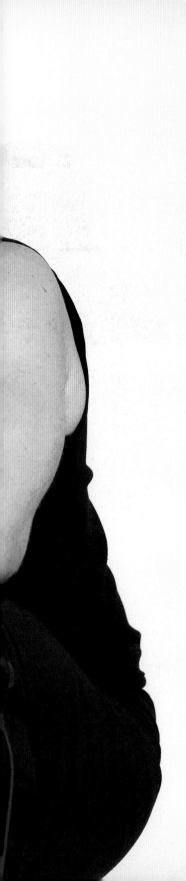

CONTENTS

FOREWORD BY
TOM HIDDLESTON

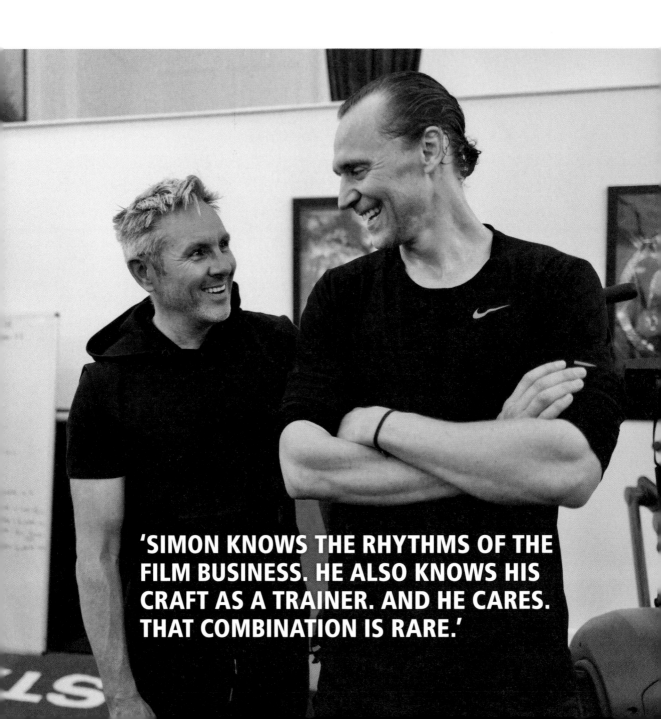

'SIMON KNOWS THE RHYTHMS OF THE FILM BUSINESS. HE ALSO KNOWS HIS CRAFT AS A TRAINER. AND HE CARES. THAT COMBINATION IS RARE.'

I didn't plan on writing about the soft furnishings in Simon's gym at Pinewood Studios. But he's got a cushion in there on a sofa – away from the equipment, where you run and lift and sweat – that's hard to ignore. I see it every time I'm in his gym – sometimes I even sit on it – and I think it encapsulates Simon's philosophy, reminding us how we should all be approaching our fitness, and life as well. It's embroidered with the words 'One Day at a Time'.

At the beginning of any project or challenge, it feels as though you're looking up at a huge mountain and you're asking yourself, 'How am I going to climb it?' All you can do, I've realized, is put one foot in front of the other. For me, the accumulation of days – the physical preparation with Simon in pre-production; the 4 a.m. workouts throughout the shoot; locking scenes and sending them off to the film editor – means I eventually have a certain amount of work in the rear-view mirror. You reach a point where the engine is warm, any nerves have dissipated and you're thinking, 'OK, I can take this one day at a time, one scene at a time'. You're doing what Simon's cushion commands.

Where do I start with Simon's qualities as a trainer? There's the precision, the diligence, the detail, the conscientiousness, the good humour, the curiosity and the encouragement. But, above all, I admire him for the care he takes. That's what makes him tremendous. Genuinely, he's so careful.

Simon knows the rhythms of the film business. He also knows his craft as a trainer. And he cares. That combination is rare. He understands how to prime actors for ninety-day shooting schedules, how to give us the skills and physical capabilities we'll need. And he always goes beyond. He takes pride in what he's doing. Every day in his gym, that care is evident.

It's not just that Simon cares about the work we're putting in, but he also cares about you as a person. He's kind and he's honest. We've worked together on several film and television productions – from *The Night Manager* and *Kong: Skull Island* to *Thor: Ragnarok* and *Loki* – and in between projects he will get in touch to see how I am. I remember an occasion when Simon was working on a Star Wars film (which I wasn't in) and he messaged me to ask whether I wanted to come into his gym for a session. It's always fun to check in with him.

Different characters, stories and productions are going to require different skills and abilities. Simon tailors my programme according to my specific needs for each role. When these projects are released, the joy, I think, for the audience is that they can get lost in the illusion and the magic. They don't need to see the strings. To ensure that it looks believable on screen, Simon helps me to be physically ready so the viewer doesn't see those strings. Some days I'll be sprinting at 3 a.m., trying to lock an outdoor scene before the sun comes up. Other days I'll be in a harness, flying through the air in front of a blue screen – perhaps falling through space or down a wormhole – and I'll need a strong core to maintain my position up there on the wire.

Simon knows I adore the freedom and the endorphin rush of running, and he has integrated that into my workouts, with warm-ups and sprints on the treadmill. But he also throws things in there that I find difficult. He breaks it all down. I use the same accumulator method that you'll read about in this book, and he puts all the exercises on a whiteboard for me. This enables me to prepare for the ones I find most challenging, as Simon has helped me to understand what my weaknesses are in the gym and also where my strengths lie.

The most intense period with Simon tends to be when you're about three or four weeks away from the first day of shooting. That's when you have the chance to push the engine a little bit, and accelerate your progression, as you don't have the constraints of filming later that day. When I'm shooting, I'm in the gym with Simon at 4 a.m., as otherwise I won't have the time to train and then go through what's known as the works – hair, make-up and costume – before the day's first take shortly after 8 a.m. Any later and you lose the chance to build the momentum of the day. Simon never complains about the early starts. We fire up the espresso machine, have our coffees and I step on the treadmill to warm up. While I'm running, Simon will be chatting to me, maybe discussing the sport from the night before, while establishing how I am, how I slept and where my energy levels are that morning.

I like working out before arriving on set as I find it gets me into the right mindset. The hardest part is the early-morning alarm. But if I'm feeling tired when I get to Simon's gym, a workout will lift me up. If I arrive feeling a bit overstimulated, a session can bring me down a little. That time with Simon creates an equilibrium. It's a routine. As I train, I've got the scene of the day in my head, so it's a kind of mental preparation, too. By the time I'm on set and we start putting the scene together, I'm already wide awake – there's oxygen in my brain and my nervous system has been stimulated. I'm reacting and listening and, I hope, collaborating in a more cohesive way with everyone else.

Simon's gym at Pinewood Studios is a collegiate place. I've seen plenty of actors in there. They appreciate that space. When actors are new to Marvel and they're training with Simon for the first time, you sometimes get the sense that

'HE HAS THE WISDOM OF KNOWING WHEN TO PUSH ME AND WHEN TO EASE OFF.'

they're thinking, 'Wow, his workouts are really intense.' Those actors are witnessing a part of the film-making process that they haven't experienced before.

But my sessions with Simon aren't always at maximum intensity. He has the wisdom of knowing when to push me and when to ease off. Perhaps I've had a huge day, shooting a scene with high emotional stakes and physicality. It's been exciting and hopefully that transmits on the screen, but there will definitely be an echo of that when I come in the next morning. Seeing that I'm knackered, Simon will say: 'We don't have to go too hard today. Let's just get moving, get the heart rate up, have a stretch and do some active recovery to get the lactic acid out of your muscles.' Simon gives me the reassurance that I don't have to go after any personal bests that day.

For me, training with Simon is a crucial part of preparing for any action role. And I know I'm not alone in thinking that Simon is a gem. Some of the best actors in the world love training with him. He's done some extraordinary work. This ten-week programme is a fantastic example of Simon's thoughtful and effective approach to fitness, and should enable lots more people to benefit from his unparalleled knowledge of what it takes to reach your physical goals.

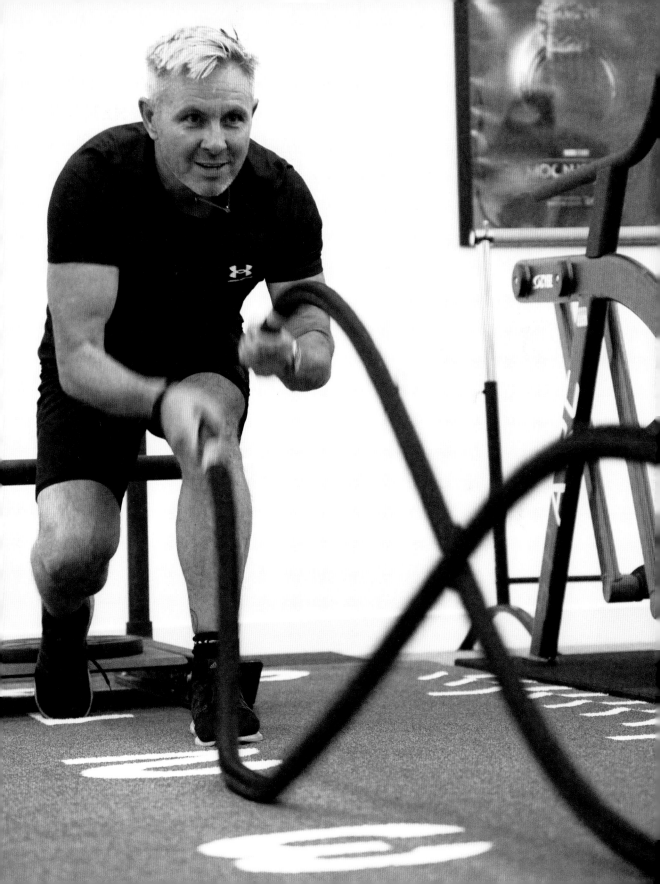

INTRODUCTION

My job as a health and fitness coach in the film industry is to support actors in their efforts to play some of cinema's most iconic, and also athletic, characters. As Tom Hiddleston wrote in his foreword, it's about ensuring that the viewers don't see the strings, but it's also about giving clients the capability to deal with the demands of shooting a movie.

In addition to working with Tom while he filmed *Loki*, *The Night Manager* and other projects, I trained Daniel Craig for his five Bond movies (from *Casino Royale* to *No Time to Die*), Chris Evans for *Captain America*, Benedict Cumberbatch for *Doctor Strange*, Bryce Dallas Howard for *Jurassic World*, John Boyega for *Star Wars*, and many others. Using my Intelligent Fitness approach, I continue to collaborate with actors at the top of their game to help them perform physically demanding roles.

My Intelligent Fitness philosophy is about training for pure performance rather than aesthetic. As I often say to the actors that I work with, aesthetic is a by-product of performance. Fitness is primarily about feelings and enjoyment; if you feel good, that's going to be reflected on the outside and how

you look, as you're going to get the consistency and continuity you need. By focusing on the mental and emotional aspects of your health and wellbeing, rather than just the physical side, you can gain a much more well-rounded and sustainable approach to fitness.

Ten weeks is not just a nice round number, but it's also typically how long I have with an actor in pre-production when I'm training them for a role. It is usually long enough to turn actors into athletes, both physically and mentally. Ten weeks is also the ideal amount of time for you to reboot your fitness using the same methods, insights and motivational advice that I give to the actors you see on screen.

FEEL AND SEE THE RESULTS

Whatever your own personal goal – which could be reducing body fat or weight, increasing muscle tissue or improving your all-round physical and mental wellbeing to feel good – this book will help you to make real progress in ten weeks. I find it takes this length of time to change habits and experience an overall progression in your fitness. Complete this programme and you'll be able to feel and see the results.

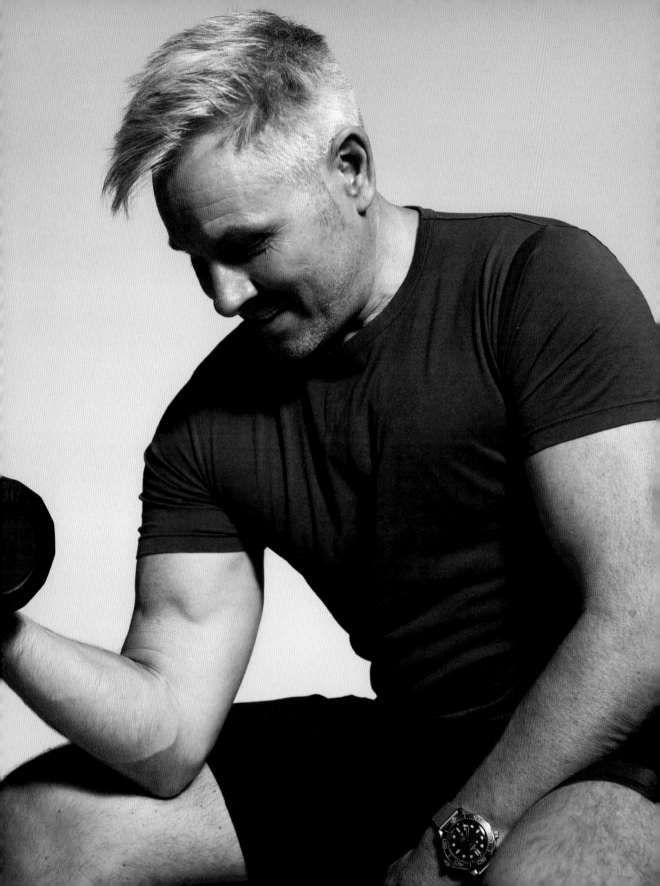

We all love a challenge. Whether you're new to fitness, or at an intermediate or advanced level, this book is for you. Maybe you've never even considered embarking upon a fitness challenge before, or perhaps you're looking to freshen up what you're doing in the gym, or to take your fitness somewhere new. Everyone's welcome. I'm giving you the structure and the easy-to-follow workout guides.

A-LIST INSPIRATION

You won't just be challenging yourself physically; you'll also be testing yourself mentally. That's why I want to provide you with the inspiration and the motivation to get you through the ten weeks, as I know how important it is to have the right mental approach. I hope that the endorsements at the start of each chapter from some of my biggest clients who have benefitted from my fitness programmes will encourage you to stick with this challenge, knowing that others have seen amazing results with my workouts.

I'm also providing you with the same tips and tricks that I give actors to ensure that you get the most out of the next ten weeks, including how to survive the notorious Week 6, when many people tend to be low on motivation. There's also a twist in Week 10, when I give you the same surprise that I spring on many of my clients at the end of their fitness programmes, which tends to shock them, but helps them to feel amazing about what they have accomplished.

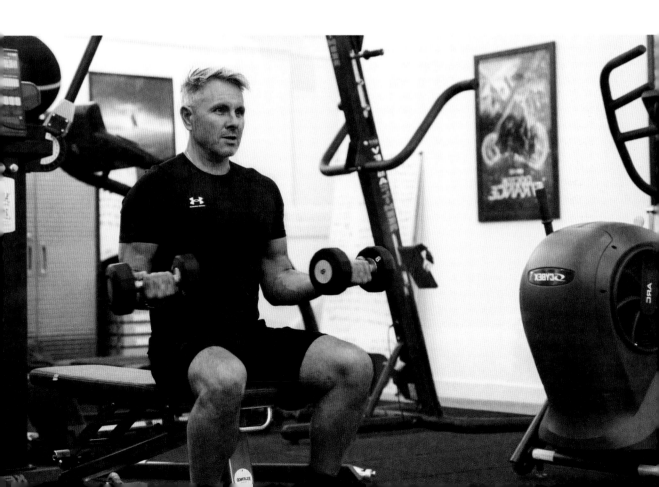

While you should be clear in your mind about why you're taking on my challenge, I encourage you not to put a number on your goal. Make your aims as broad as possible. If you're looking to lose weight, for instance, don't have a precise figure in mind, because if you fall a little short you're going to think you've failed or underachieved, and you won't give yourself any credit for what you have accomplished. If your goal is enhancing your mental wellbeing, and you're hoping to supercharge how you feel, move and breathe, those aren't things you can easily measure.

GET READY TO GLOW

Friends and family can be very supportive, encouraging you through some of the tough moments, so it can be helpful to let them know that you're about to embark on this fitness challenge. It's also good to have a training partner alongside you, or someone else who is like-minded and on their own fitness journey, because working out as part of a team can be a great motivator. But maybe don't announce it to the world that you're doing a challenge. The greatest compliment you're going to get at the end of this experience – and the thought of this could be a significant motivation – is when somebody you haven't seen for ten weeks says to you: 'Wow, you're like a completely different person.' You'll have a real glow about you. You'll look different. You may have better posture, more positive energy and more bounce in your step with a sense of achievement and fulfilment, as well as the physiological effects. And although no one can see it, everything inside your body will be functioning more efficiently.

THE ACCUMULATOR METHOD

In my first book, *Intelligent Fitness*, I introduced you to the accumulator or 5–2 method that I use with the majority of my clients, as I believe that will give you the best results in the shortest period of time. That's also how your workouts will be organized over the next ten weeks. Every workout has five exercises and includes short bursts of cardio (between two and five minutes, depending on how far you are into the programme).

Each workout will be structured like this:

Exercise 1
Cardio
Exercise 1
Exercise 2
Cardio
Exercise 1
Exercise 2
Exercise 3
Cardio
Exercise 1
Exercise 2
Exercise 3
Exercise 4
Cardio
Exercise 1
Exercise 2
Exercise 3
Exercise 4
Exercise 5
Cardio

Splitting up the cardio, doing short bursts between exercises rather than in one large block, helps to keep your workout dynamic and interesting. As you're constantly moving from one activity to another, you don't ever have time to get bored. You're having to think about what's coming up next and that can help distract you from how hard you're working. Carrying out your cardio in bursts is much easier to deal with. I feel as though you can do anything for two minutes (or up to five minutes towards the end of the challenge), but if you're faced with the thought of attempting twenty minutes or so of cardio, you might not think you can manage it.

Some people think they're cardio people and don't want to touch the weights. Others see themselves as weights people and don't like cardio. But this method brings everything together, giving you a balanced workout.

Look out for the weeks when I increase the amount of cardio between exercises – when I think you're ready, I'll add another minute (find your coloured accumulator instruction box at the start of every new week!). In Week 1, for instance, you'll be doing two minutes of cardio between the exercises, which is 5–2. But by Week 9, which is the most intense

FROM RUNNING TO GETTING ON THE BIKE TO THE ROWING MACHINE, CARDIO IS ANYTHING WHICH ELEVATES YOUR HEART RATE.

stage of the programme, you'll be at 5–5, with five minutes of cardio. There's some choice, though, as it's up to you which type of cardio you do. From running to getting on the bike to the rowing machine, cardio is anything which elevates your heart rate.

My clients like these workouts as they're fast and efficient, with each one taking about thirty to forty minutes (they become a little longer as I increase the cardio). You also have your bolt-ons, such as your ten-minute activation or warm-up, and then ten or fifteen minutes of stretching at the end, but you should still be able to easily fit this into your day.

THE RHYTHM OF THE WEEK
Every week has a similar rhythm to it. Monday is legs day (I know everyone hates doing legs and that's why it's good to do that on a Monday, because then it's over and done with for the week), Tuesday is upper body, Wednesday is dynamic stretching, Thursday is core, Friday is full body, Saturday is active sport, and Sunday is wellness and recovery. I've organized the week in that order – the same order I use with my clients – as that allows you to rest muscle groups and recover so you are fresh for your next workout, helping you to progress your fitness.

FEEL-GOOD FRIDAY
Friday should be a feel-good day. I want to give you a rush of endorphins as you go into the weekend. That's why on each Friday, I've pooled some of the exercises you would have done earlier in the week in your Monday legs workout and your Tuesday upper-body workout. I take the same approach with actors as that means they will be doing exercises with which they're familiar. You're not having to figure out new exercises because your body already knows

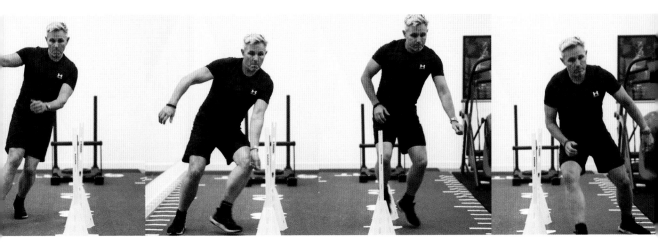

the patterns. It's Familiar Friday, too: your workout should be easier, faster and more efficient, and likely to make you feel good. You're in touch with every single part of your body, which is great for both your wellbeing and your fitness.

MENTAL STIMULATION

I've designed the workouts so you can easily make progress with your fitness. Every week, the exercises have been tweaked and adapted from the ones the week before, so your body is following similar patterns but you're making important incremental progress as you move through the programme. As you're constantly building, you're more likely to feel motivated and that's going to help to give you the consistency you need for this to be sustainable.

Changing it up each week also stops you from getting bored. There are a few people who are perfectly happy doing the same exercises week after week, as they know exactly where they are with them and they like what the routine does for their mind and body. But most of us want a little variety, as that provides some mental stimulation and helps

to maintain interest and engagement. Another advantage of a more varied programme is that, while you're hitting the same muscle groups each week, you're doing it slightly differently and that aids your progression.

At the same time, you don't always want change and variety. You'll see that I have designed the programme so you do the same dynamic stretching and core exercises in Weeks 1–3, with another block for Weeks 4–6 and a third for Weeks 7–9. (I won't ruin the surprise by telling you what I have planned for you in Week 10.) That should help you to achieve the best results.

Go ahead and test yourself. See the results you can achieve during the ten weeks. Like anything in life, you'll only get out what you put in. I've designed this challenge to be easily repeatable and adaptable, to be used whenever you want to refresh your fitness. You can come back to this book again and again, taking things to a new level each time.

HOW TO USE THIS BOOK

It's important that you know exactly what's coming up when you're training, which is why I like to put a client's workout on a whiteboard in the gym. While I can't be with you in person, I hope that the way I have designed the 10-Week Intelligent Fitness Challenge makes it easy to follow and understand. Don't be afraid to take this book into the gym, or wherever you're training, and to treat it as if it's your version of an Intelligent Fitness whiteboard. To remind you of what you're doing each day, and also so you can look at each week at a glance, I've included a grid at the end of each chapter that shows all the exercises.

STRUCTURE AND FORM IS KEY

If you're going to get the most out of this challenge, please make sure that you go through the weeks chronologically, rather than jumping around and mixing up the order, or even skipping weeks. I want you to feel as though you're getting fitter, but if you're swapping or missing weeks you won't get that same sense of progression. I would also advise you to follow the step-by-step instructions for each of the exercises as closely as you can, looking at the

form in the images, as that will help to ensure you're training the muscles correctly and safely, which is going to reduce your chance of injury and setbacks.

Within the structure of this challenge, there is still plenty of scope for personal choice and flexibility, not least because you can pick the cardio you do for the accumulator method, and you're also free on Saturdays and Sundays to find your own way to get active, recover and fill up your wellness jar. When you reach weeks 7–9, I've given you some extra options for your Thursday core workouts, which should provide you with additional variety and stimulation.

If you've never done a fitness programme before, you might well be wondering how you're going to fit training into your day. One tip is to train early in the morning, because then you're more likely to do the session rather than dropping it later in the day if something comes up at work or in your personal life (though, as I write in Chapter 7, you mustn't ever feel guilty about missing a workout for a good reason, as that's life and things can crop up unexpectedly).

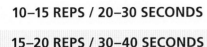
MAKE THE CHALLENGE WORK FOR YOU

This book is for people of all abilities: for those who are just getting started with fitness, or others who are at an intermediate or advanced level. Each of the workouts, even each of the exercises, can be done at three different levels by varying the rep range. You will see the colour-coded bars at the top of the page for every new week (like the ones above) as a reminder of how many reps you should be doing, or the period of time over which you should repeat them (some of us prefer to measure in time rather than reps) depending on the intensity you require.

When you're a few weeks into the challenge, you might find that you want to push on from beginner to intermediate or from intermediate to advanced. The three different levels will also allow you to revisit this programme, offering you a fresh and stimulating challenge every time.

CHOOSING YOUR WEIGHTS

We always overestimate what we can lift. When selecting your weights, think of the maximum you believe you could do the exercise with. Now go 25 per cent lighter and you'll probably be bang on the money. Always use a weight that's within your capability. Perhaps you do a few reps with one weight and you feel as though you can't possibly finish the set. There's no harm in dropping to a lower weight in order to complete the full set of reps. If you're doing the challenge for a second, third or fourth time, you'll no doubt find you can use heavier weights than you did the first time.

TIPS FOR EACH DAY OF THE WEEK

As each week has the same structure and rhythm – with a legs workout on the Monday, an upper-body workout on the Tuesday, and so on – here are some pointers to help you throughout the challenge:

Tips for Monday: legs

If you feel as though you're getting cramp, your muscles are tighter than usual or you're fatiguing too quickly, stop to hydrate and stretch. Listen to your body before carrying on. Always try to have soft knees, which is when you keep the emphasis on the muscles rather than on the joints. As soon as you lock out your knees, you will put all your weight and pressure on the joints, but you need to be targeting the muscles as that will allow you to get stronger.

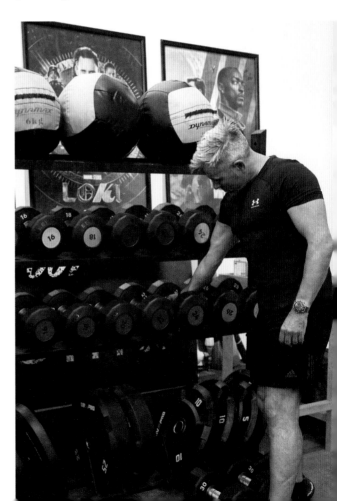

Tips for Tuesday: upper body

Always ensure you have the full range of motion, and you're doing the rep from the start to the finish, rather than a short rep. You'll then be maintaining tension on the muscle tissue for as long as possible, which will give you optimal results. Keep your knees soft as that allows you to be springy.

Tips for Wednesday: dynamic stretching (and also for post-workout stretching on any day)

The most important thing about stretching is maintaining control, which you can do through tempo and flow. You're in total command of your body, including your breathing. Breathe in through your nose, making sure you fill your lungs. Hold that breath and then breathe out through your mouth in a controlled manner, exhaling all the air. Hold the stretch until you can feel a comfortable pain. Keep on holding it until the soreness disappears and then add 10 per cent to the stretch, which should give you a bearable discomfort. Wait for that to disappear and then add another 10 per cent. Now ease off slowly. Control is key because the negative element of a stretch is just as important as the positive one. That's all part of the stretch, and you're not allowing gravity to do the work for you.

Tips for Thursday: core

The core is the most overtrained part of the body. People seem to think that more is more when training their core muscles, and they fatigue those muscles every day rather than letting them recover and allowing adaptation (changes in your muscles as they adjust to the exercises) to take its course. You have to treat your core muscles like any other in your body. Perhaps you don't realize that your core muscles are engaged when doing legs and upper-body exercises, so you'll be training them on other days as well as on Thursdays. Don't be afraid to take

a break during a set, but always resume and get to the desired number of reps (something to bear in mind on all days and not just Thursdays).

Tips for Friday: full body

Don't be alarmed if your heart rate is more elevated on a Friday – you're asking more of your cardiovascular system, which is pumping more blood and oxygen all around the body, looking after every single muscle group. But your heart can work harder than you might imagine. A general rule of thumb is that your maximum heart rate should be 220 beats per minute minus your age. Instead of worrying, enjoy that feeling of working hard as it's going to give you an endorphin high.

Tips for Saturday: active sport

Do something you enjoy – this could be going for a run or a bike ride, trekking, playing tennis or having a very active day with your family. Move your body how you want to. But get active for at least an hour. While Monday to Friday is structured, your Saturday should be freer and be more about escapism. Make sure it's enjoyable. Maybe the reason you're training is that you want to be fitter to do the sport or activity you love, and Saturday is the chance to make the most of your new capability and energy. Or perhaps you could take the opportunity to try something new. Improving your fitness will boost your confidence, which will encourage you to do unfamiliar things. The more capable you feel, the more likely you are to sample new sports and activities, which offers stimulation and helps to keep you interested in your fitness.

Tips for Sunday: wellness and recovery

This is the day for filling up your wellness jar. Go for a walk along the beach, by a lake or river, or take a ramble through the countryside. I say this all the time to actors – get outside as there's nothing better than being in nature, especially during the summer months. It's fantastic for your mental health and wellbeing as you're stimulating all your senses.

Recovery isn't just about getting treatment on a massage table (though you may wish to do that). Maybe have a lie-in, meditate, do some yoga or Pilates, or have a sauna or go for a steam. Recovery is key to every fitness programme because if you don't do it properly after each training session, you won't make any progress. You might wish to use contactless percussion tools, electrical stimulation aids and cold-water therapy, or even treat yourself to a massage or an appointment with an osteopath or chiropractor.

Sunday is also a chance to give yourself a pat on the back for completing a week and to be reflective about how much effort you put into it – was it 70, 80 or 90 per cent, or did you stick to the programme completely? Can you give 100 per cent next week?

WEEKLY ROUND-UP

Look out for the grid at the end of each chapter, which shows all your exercises for the week on one double-page spread for those of you using the book in the gym. I've also included some weekly tips on nutrition and wellbeing that you can bear in mind as you adjust to a new week's workout.

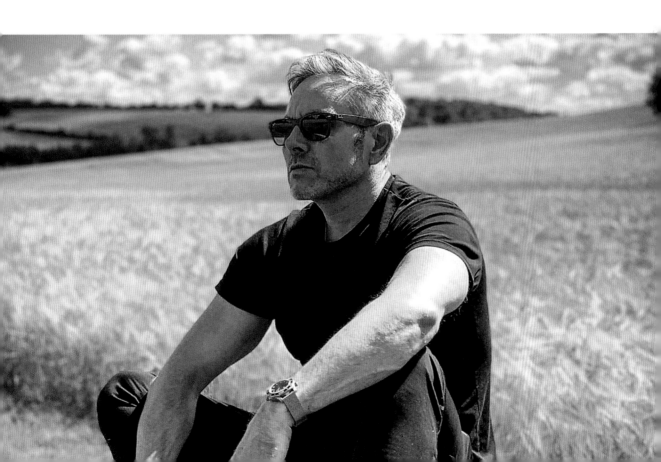

PRE- AND POST-WORKOUT

WARM-UP

Before you start your workout, do whatever activation makes you feel good. If you look at the physiology of the 'warm-up', nothing really warms up. You're not really raising your core temperature. So, although the effects aren't as great as you might imagine them to be, what you are doing is preparing yourself mentally for the task ahead – switching your brain into activity mode.

It's important to recognize that everyone is different and what works for others might not necessarily help you to prepare for training. But whatever you do, don't overload the muscles during a stretch session because then you won't get the most out of yourself during the actual workout. You might find that it helps to review the details of your next-day workout the night before, and think about what you might do in terms of a warm-up beforehand, as this will allow you to visualize what's ahead and get into the right mindset.

POST-WORKOUT

Stretching after your workout feels good, and it also signals to your body and mind that the workout is over. Your heart rate is coming down, you're in a more rested state and you're preparing for the day ahead.

Coming up are some stretches to do after a legs workout on a Monday, an upper-body session on a Tuesday and a core workout on a Thursday. (Because your Wednesday workout involves dynamic stretching, there's no need to do any more stretching at the end of this day.) For variety, you might also want to do some of the stretches that I've chosen later in the book for the dynamic stretching workouts on Wednesdays. After a full-body workout on a Friday, you can do any combination of Monday's leg stretches and Tuesday's upper-body stretches. In addition to stretching after a workout, feel free to stop between exercises for a stretch.

MONDAY
LEG STRETCHES

STANDING CALF STRETCH

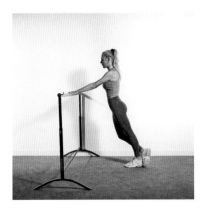 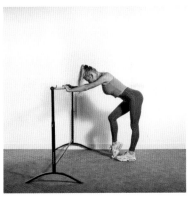 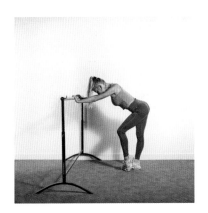

Place your palms against the wall, or hold onto a bar, and put one leg behind the other. Dip your hips forward while keeping your front heel on the ground, stretching your calf. Return to the start position and place both feet on the ground. Pedal your feet for a few seconds – this means keeping the toes of both feet on the ground and raising one heel off the floor at a time, alternating between the two. Now begin the stretch on your other calf.

GLUTES STRETCH

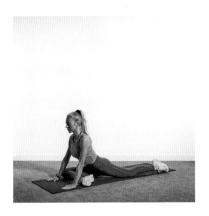 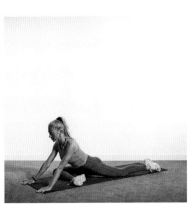

With your palms shoulder-width apart on the floor in front of you, extend one leg behind you and bring the other up with the knee bent at 90 degrees. Push your palms out in front of you a little more and feel the stretch in your glutes.

HAMSTRING STRETCH

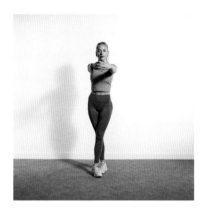 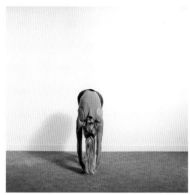

Put one leg over the other, locking out the rear hamstring, putting the emphasis on that muscle, and lean as far forward as you can. Switch legs and repeat on the other side.

ADAPTED DOWNWARD DOG WITH CALF STRETCH

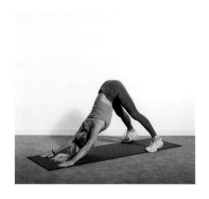 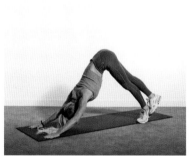

Get into the downward dog yoga position, with your feet and palms on the ground around shoulder-width apart, and your legs as straight as possible. Cross one leg over the other, resting it on the Achilles tendon, and feel the stretch through the calf. Repeat with the other leg.

POSTERIOR CHAIN STRETCH

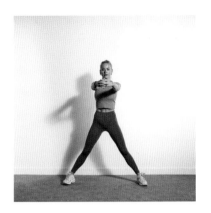 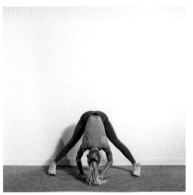

Stand with your feet a little wider than shoulder-width apart, your knees locked and your hands together. Lean forward as far as you can, aiming to touch the floor (though don't be concerned if you're not flexible enough to reach all the way). You should be feeling a comfortable stretch in your hamstrings. You could also add some bounce.

STRETCHING ENCOURAGES BLOOD FLOW INTO THE AREA YOU'RE TARGETING AND BOOSTS OXYGEN LEVELS IN YOUR BODY.

UPPER BODY STRETCHES

CHEST STRETCH

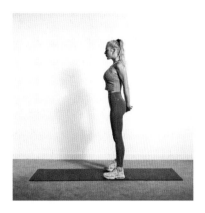 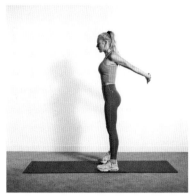

Standing with your feet shoulder-width apart, put your arms behind you, clasping your hands together. Lift your arms so you feel a stretch through your chest.

SHOULDER STRETCH

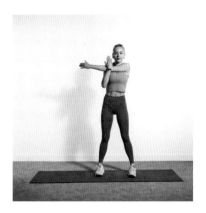 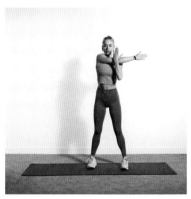

Bring one arm across your chest. Put your other arm over the top of the first arm and squeeze towards your chest. Now repeat on the other side. This stretch will keep your shoulders supple, helps to avoid injury and is also great for posture.

CORE STRETCHES

COBRA

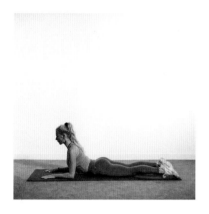 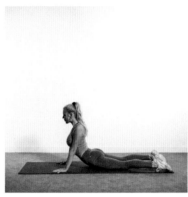

Lie face down with your toes pointing behind you and your forearms on the floor shoulder-width apart. Bring your chest up.

For a more intense stretch, push up onto your palms with your chin slightly raised.

SIDE OBLIQUES STRETCH

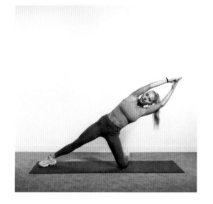

You're down on your left knee, with your right leg out to the side, and your right hand and arm going over your head. You should feel the stretch down your side obliques and your intercostals (rib muscles). You're also getting a slight stretch of the hamstring and, depending on the foot position, your abductor muscle. Now switch to the other side, getting down on your right knee.

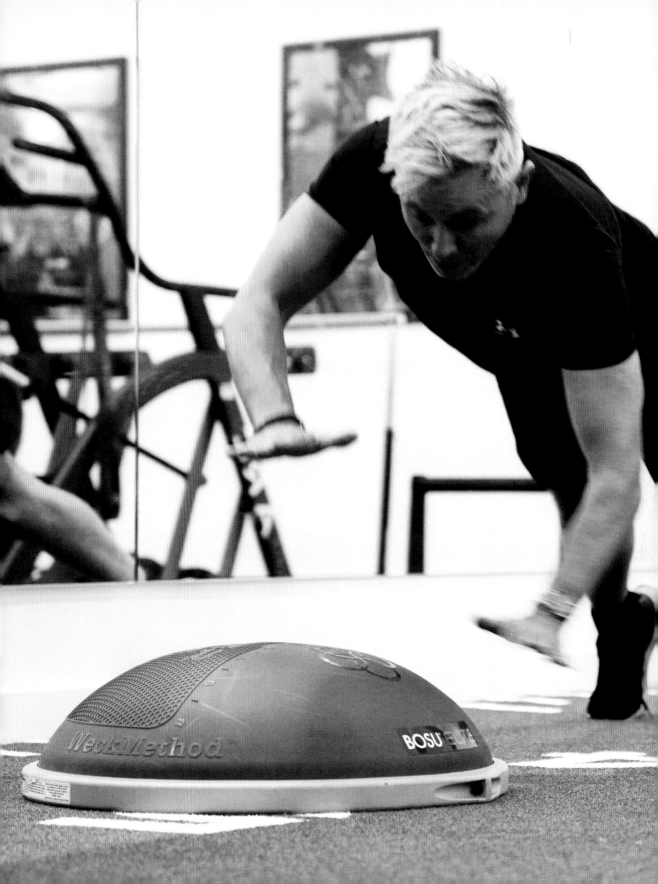

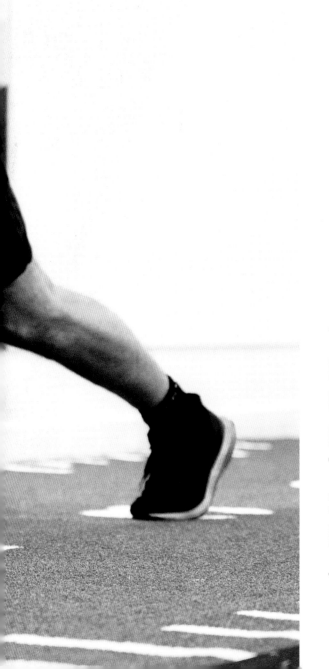

WEEK 1

'IF YOU'VE BEEN LOOKING FOR A PROGRAMME THAT IS AS CLEAR AS THE RESULTS ARE SUSTAINABLE, LOOK NO FURTHER!'

John Krasinski

GETTING STARTED

Starting slowly is actually the quickest way to get to where you want to be. Go out too fast and too hard at the beginning of a fitness challenge and you'll risk demotivating yourself before you've even begun.

ACCUMULATOR: 5–2

FINDING YOUR OWN RHYTHM

When I'm preparing actors for a movie, I don't need to motivate them in the first week as they're already engaged and energized. If anything, I might end up doing the opposite – they'll possibly be overenthusiastic and I'll be encouraging them to ease off a little so that they don't exhaust themselves too early on in their new programme. Enthusiasm is an amazing tool in fitness but, as I'm often telling clients, you need to learn how to channel that energy and adopt a more measured and sustainable approach to your fitness. If you're punishing yourself in Week 1, I guarantee that you won't last until Week 10.

In these first few days, you're figuring out your rhythm and pace, and discovering how much you're willing to give. While you need a high level of commitment to get through this challenge, you can take that too far and give too much in the initial stages. If your fitness journey and your rate of progression is going to be sustainable, it's important that you don't put *all* your energy and enthusiasm into your fitness. There will be other areas of your life that you'll also need to be focusing on over the next ten weeks, such as your work and your family.

DON'T OVERLOAD

You're starting to break old habits and create new ones. But if you make lots of change in the first week, you'll almost certainly find that it's too much to adjust to. It's a delicate process. It's almost like playing hide-and-seek with your body and your brain – they love consistency and you don't want them to notice that you're making these fitness transitions as you might find they then rebel against you. Mentally, you only have so much space to deal with the everyday, and if you're constantly thinking about exercise your brain will be overloaded and you'll be mentally fatigued the whole time, which will have a detrimental effect on what you feel you can handle the next day in terms of working out. That can stop you in your tracks before you've really set off, so be sensible.

Exercise, and making adjustments to your lifestyle, shouldn't be difficult. You never want a fitness programme to overwhelm you. Then it becomes complicated and seems like a slog, and you'll soon ditch it. Ideally, once you introduce exercise into your daily routine, it should feel like a natural part of your life. In my experience, you should drip-feed the changes over the next ten weeks in addition to the exercises I'm setting. Maybe in Week 1, make a small, simple change such as getting into the habit of always drinking a glass of water first thing in the morning and then last thing at night, as that will enhance your hydration. You're starting these habits and letting them grow and build. Once you've mastered one, you'll be ready to introduce another to your life. But never believe that you should be sorting out everything to do with your health and wellness, including hydration and nutrition, in Week 1.

BE REALISTIC

Part of not going out too fast is pitching your expectations at the right level. When you're starting

> ## WEEK 1 KIT LIST
> **BAND**
> **BAR AND WEIGHTS**
> **BENCH**
> **BOX**
> **DUMBBELLS**
> **KETTLEBELL, PLATE OR DUMBBELL**
> **ROLLER**

anything that's new and fresh, always set the bar low in the short term and then you'll feel as though you're achieving at a high level. If you set the bar too high, you probably won't get there and you'll imagine you're constantly failing. In Week 1, you might be doing many or all of these exercises for the first time. There's a lot to learn and you're educating yourself, you're starting one or two new habits and you're thinking about how you're going to get to Week 10. That should be your focus; not trying to blitz Week 1.

DON'T BE TOO HARD ON YOURSELF IN THE FIRST WEEK – GETTING STARTED IS THE TOUGHEST PART.

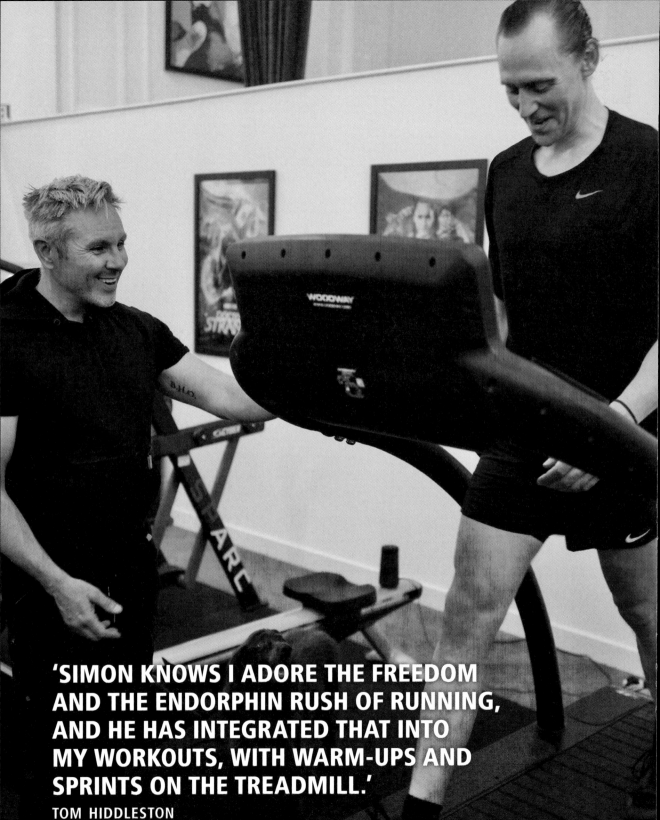

'SIMON KNOWS I ADORE THE FREEDOM AND THE ENDORPHIN RUSH OF RUNNING, AND HE HAS INTEGRATED THAT INTO MY WORKOUTS, WITH WARM-UPS AND SPRINTS ON THE TREADMILL.'

TOM HIDDLESTON

LEGS

	10–15 REPS / 20–30 SECONDS
	15–20 REPS / 30–40 SECONDS
	20–25 REPS / 40–50 SECONDS

EXERCISE 1: SQUAT

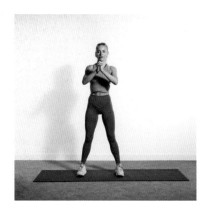
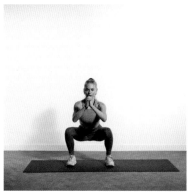

Stand with your feet shoulder-width apart, your toes pointing slightly outwards. Lower yourself down until your knees are at 90 degrees and hold that position for a count of four. Push up through your heels to return to the start position.

EXERCISE 2: BAND MATRIX

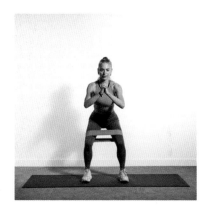
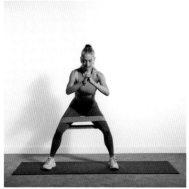
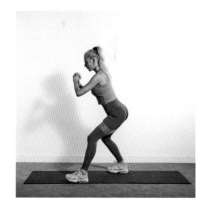

With a band just above your knees, stand with your feet shoulder-width apart and bend your knees slightly. Clasp your hands together in front of you while focusing straight ahead. Start with sidesteps, repeating small squat steps to the right and left, the number of reps dependent on what level you're exercising at. Maintaining tension in the band, put your left foot forward around 10 inches or 25 centimetres, move your right foot forward the same distance, before moving your left foot back followed by your right.

EXERCISE 3: LUNGE

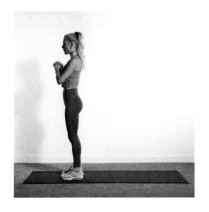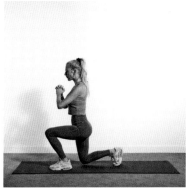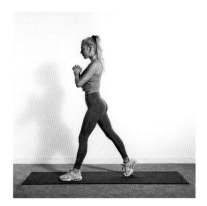

Stand with your feet shoulder-width apart. Lunge back, dropping your rear leg until your knee kisses the floor. Push upwards, returning to the start position. Swap the legs over, doing the same number of reps on each side.

EXERCISE 4: BOX STEP

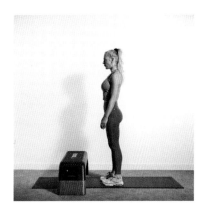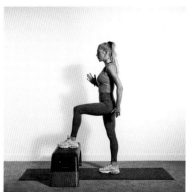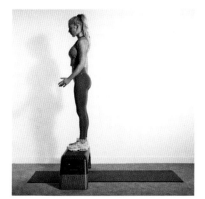

Stand 10 inches or 25 centimetres back from the box with your feet shoulder-width apart and your arms by your sides. Step onto the box with both feet and then step back down, leading with the opposite leg. For safety reasons, don't jump down – you won't benefit from doing this. After reps, start with the opposite leg and repeat.

EXERCISE 5: HIP THRUST

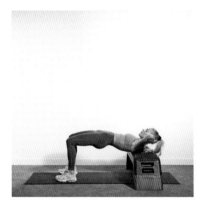 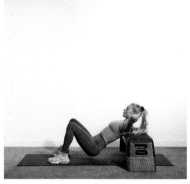

Lie back, with your shoulder blades on the bench, your knees at 90 degrees and your feet shoulder-width apart. Lower your glutes until they're about an inch or 2.5 centimetres off the ground. With control, return to the start position while contracting the glutes.

WAKE UP YOUR BODY AND GET IT MOVING. YOU'RE PREPARING FOR THE CHALLENGE AHEAD.

UPPER BODY

EXERCISE 1: PUSH-UP

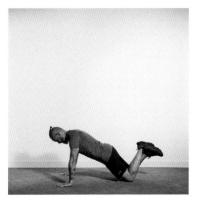
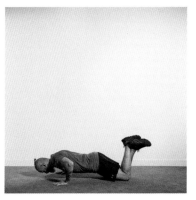

Place your hands on the ground shoulder-width apart. If this exercise is new to you, you might find it easier to rest your knees on the ground and cross your ankles behind you. Lower yourself down until your elbows are at 90 degrees. Push up and return to the start position, breathing out on exertion.

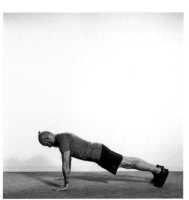
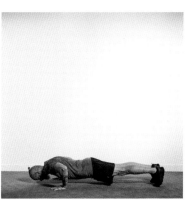

For extra intensity, take your knees off the ground and straighten your legs, keep a neutral back and neck, and do the same movement. For a more advanced version, do this exercise holding two dumbbells – this will straighten your wrists and allow you to lower yourself further.

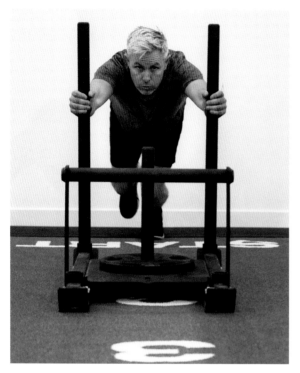
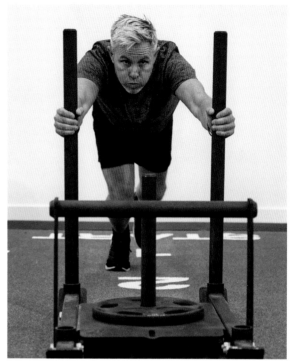
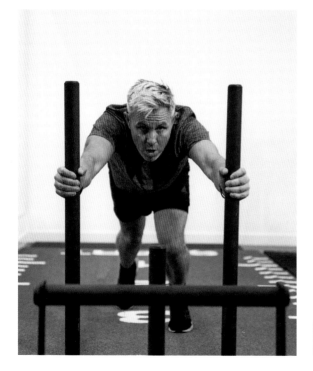
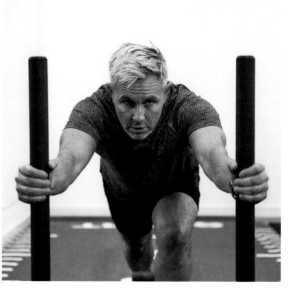

EXERCISE 2: SHOULDER MATRIX

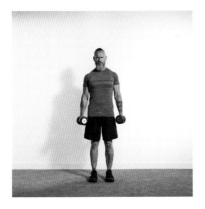 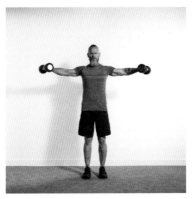

For the lateral raises, lift the dumbbells to the side with slightly bent elbows, so they are level with your shoulders. Return to the start position and transition from lateral raises into a shoulder press.

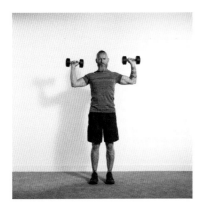 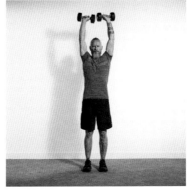

Hold the dumbbells so that your arms are at 90 degrees on either side and the dumbbells are about 6 inches or 15 centimetres away from your ears. Raise the dumbbells into the air and then bring them together so they gently kiss. Bring them back down so your elbows and arms are at 90 degrees once again.

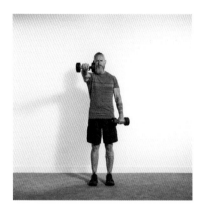
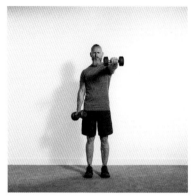

Transition into alternate forward raises. Hold the dumbbells so they are touching your thighs and then lift one dumbbell up with a slightly bent elbow to shoulder height before returning to the start position. Repeat on the other side.

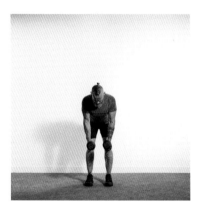
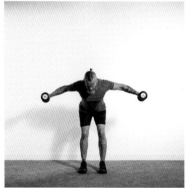

Transition into a bent-over row. Have a little bend in your knees. Maintain a neutral spine, back and neck. The dumbbells are dangling in front of you below chest height. With a slight bend in your elbows, retract the dumbbells so they are level with your shoulders and then return to the start position.

EXERCISE 3: ARMS MATRIX

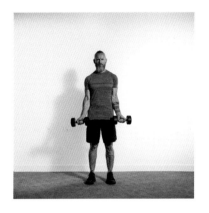 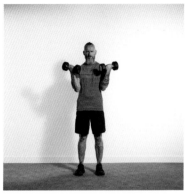 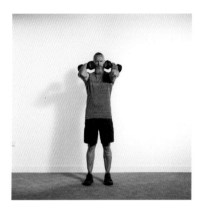

Hold a dumbbell in each hand so they are about 6 inches or
15 centimetres away from your legs, with your palms facing away from
your body. Slowly raise your dumbbells up to shoulder height, bending
your elbows. Lift your elbows a couple of inches or 5 centimetres higher
for extra pressure and then return to the start position.

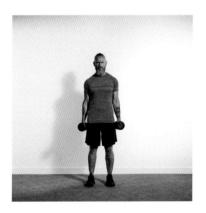 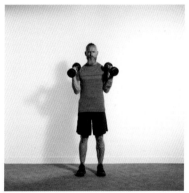

Change the hand position so your palms are now facing your body and
the dumbbells are close to your legs. Curl the dumbbells up to shoulder
height and then, with a little tip of the elbows, return to the start position.

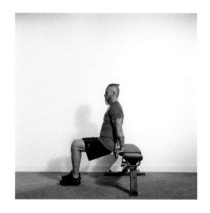 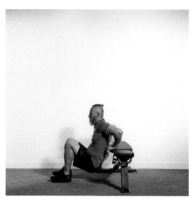

You'll need a bench for triceps dips. You should almost be sitting on your hands, with your fingers coming off the edge of the bench. Lower yourself down until your elbows are at 90 degrees. Return to the start position.

ENJOY THE CHALLENGE BUT DON'T PUNISH YOURSELF – OTHERWISE YOU WON'T LAST UNTIL WEEK 10.

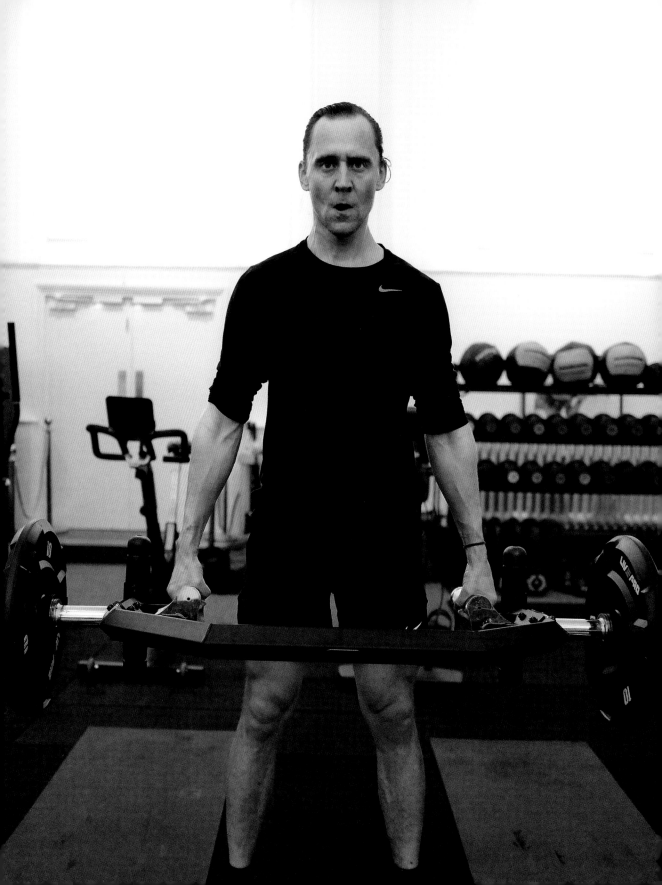

EXERCISE 4: BARBELL ROW

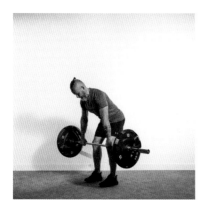 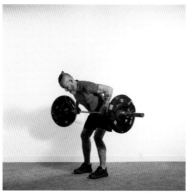

After adding the right amount of weight to suit your ability, place the barbell in front of you. Bend your knees a little. Keeping a neutral back, use an overhand grip to clasp the bar and bring it up to your knees. Slide the bar up your thighs into your waist, retracting the back and squeezing the lats. Return to the start position near your knees.

EXERCISE 5: CLEAN AND PRESS

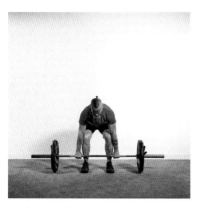 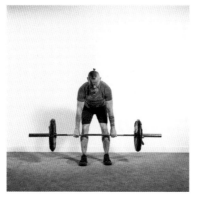

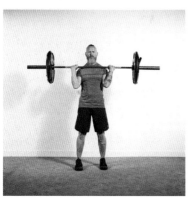 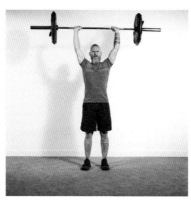

Put a moderate weight on the bar. Stand in front of the bar with your feet shoulder-width apart. Use an overhand grip, and keep a neutral back and neck. As you lift the bar up, it will naturally brush your thighs. With your elbows high, flip the bar over so that your palms are facing the ceiling. Raise the bar until your elbows are locked out or straight. Return the bar to your chest and allow it to flip back to your thighs and back down to the ground.

DYNAMIC STRETCHING

10–15 REPS / 20–30 SECONDS	
15–20 REPS / 30–40 SECONDS	
20–25 REPS / 40–50 SECONDS	

EXERCISE 1: BEAR CRAWL INTO PIGEON

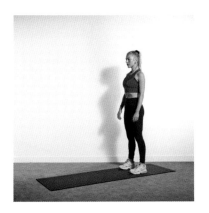 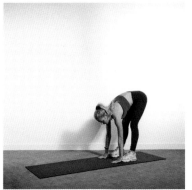 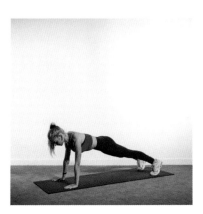

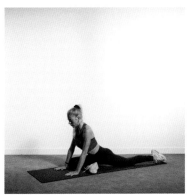 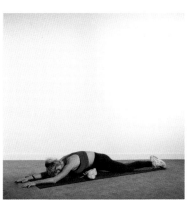 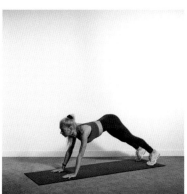

Stand with your feet shoulder-width apart. Bend down, pivoting from the hip until your hands hit the floor in front of you. Crawl out until you are in a plank position. Move one leg forward, placing your knee on the ground at a 90-degree angle and steadily moving down onto your forearms. As that stretch starts to ease, extend your fingers and lower your chest to your knee reaching your hands forward so your arms are flat on the ground with your leg underneath you at 45 degrees. With your hands shoulder-width apart, push yourself up and bring your leg back to the original starting position. Crawl your hands back incrementally, and slowly return to the standing position. Repeat on the other side.

EXERCISE 2: BEAR CRAWL INTO COBRA

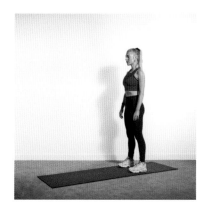 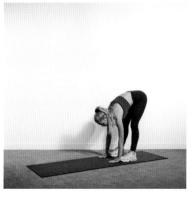 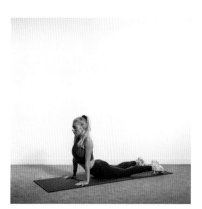

Stand with your feet shoulder-width apart and your hands by your sides.
Bend down gradually, pivoting from the hip until your hands hit the floor
in front of you. Crawl out until you are flat in a plank position. Go into
the cobra position, where your chest comes forward and your hips are
on the ground. Return to the start position.

EXERCISE 3: SIT-UP WITH LUMBAR TWIST

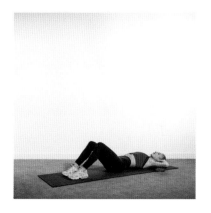 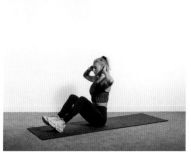 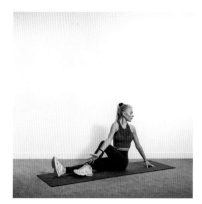

Lie on your back with your feet on the floor, your legs bent with raised
knees and your hands behind your ears. Raise yourself up and do a
regular sit-up, but as you reach the end point, put both legs flat on the
ground and then bend one leg so that the ankle is on the outside of the
opposite raised knee. Put your elbow on the outside of your raised knee
and twist until you feel a slight stretch in your lower back. Return to the
start position and repeat on the other side.

EXERCISE 4: SIDE CRAB

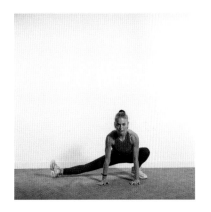 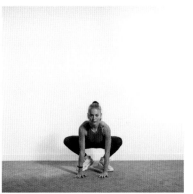 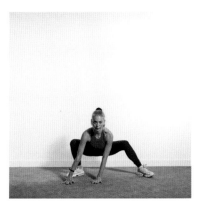

Squat down with your hands in front of you. Crawl to the side in that squatted position, and then shoot your leg out in the same direction, before returning to the squat position. Now crawl in the other direction, extend your leg and then come back to the squat position after shifting to the left and right.

ANIMALISTIC EXERCISES LIKE THIS HELP YOUR BODY MOVE MORE NATURALLY.

EXERCISE 5: PLYOMETRIC WITH A JUMP

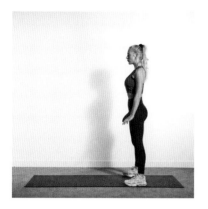 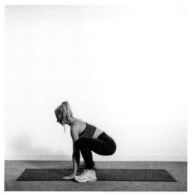 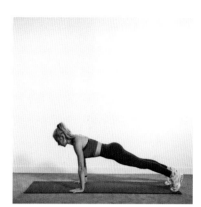

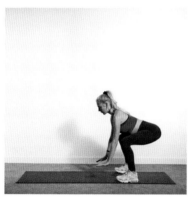 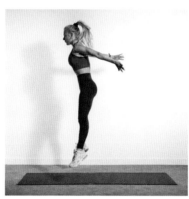

Stand with your feet shoulder-width apart and then squat down until your palms touch the floor. Your legs shoot out together behind you into a plank position. Quickly bring your legs back, with your knees to your chest, and then jump up in the air. Return to the squat position, palms on the floor.

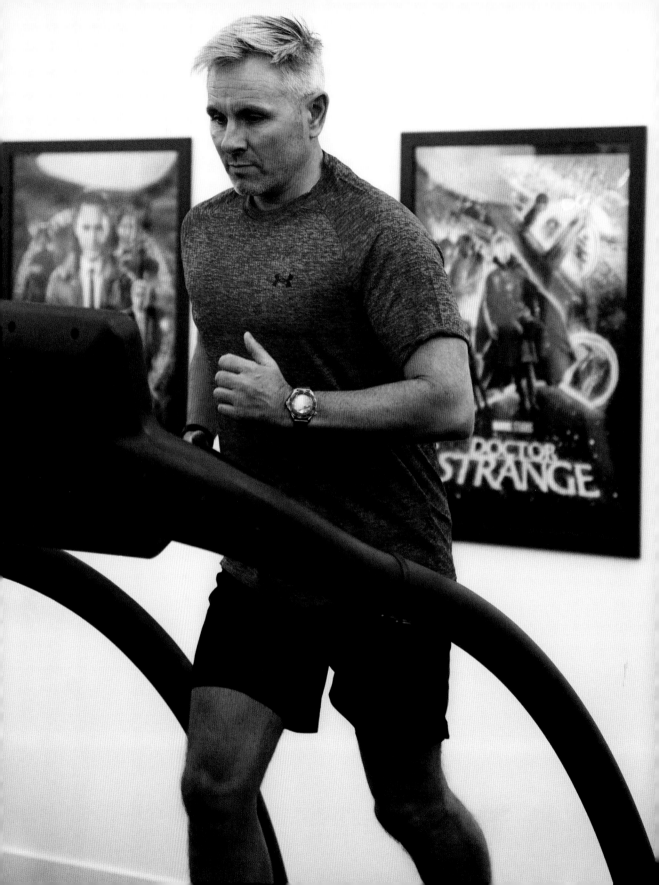

CORE

EXERCISE 1: PLANK TO PIKE TO SHOULDER TAPS

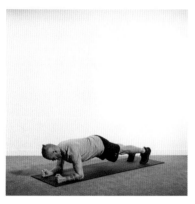
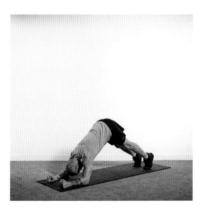

Get into the plank position, facing the floor with your hips off the ground, your forearms on the floor, and with tight glutes, a tight core and neutral back. Raise your glutes into the air into the pike position. Return to the start position.

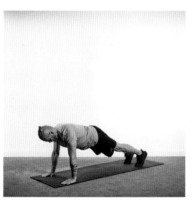
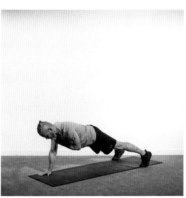

Transition into an extended plank – you're on the palms of your hands, which are fully extended as if in a push-up position. Lift your left arm, touch your right shoulder and return your arm to the floor. Now do the same on the other side.

EXERCISE 2: CRUNCHES, LEG RAISES AND HEEL TAPS

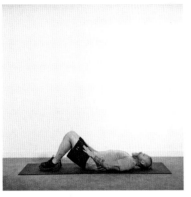
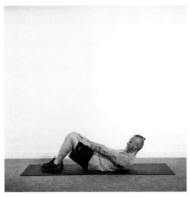

For the crunches, lie on your back with your feet flat on the floor shoulder-width apart. Place your hands on your thighs. Slide your hands to the tops of your knees while maintaining a neutral back. Return to the start position.

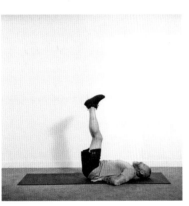
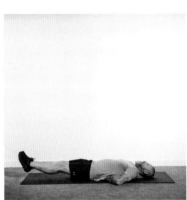

For the leg raises, lie on your back and move your legs up to an angle of 90 degrees. Slide your hands under your coccyx to support your lower back. Slowly bring your legs back down to 6 inches or 15 centimetres off the floor. Keep your abdominals tight and engaged, with your lower back pressed into the ground. Return to the start position.

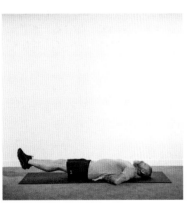
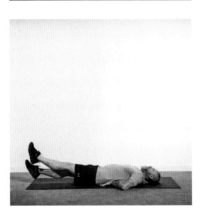

For the heel taps, stay on your back. Slide your hands under your coccyx again. Lift both legs 6 inches or 15 centimetres off the ground, keeping them straight. Next, lower one heel to 2 inches or 5 centimetres above the ground, lift and then repeat on the other side, alternating between the two legs.

EXERCISE 3: ABDOMINAL ROLLOUT WITH A ROLLER

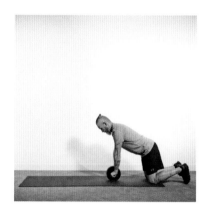 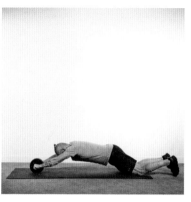 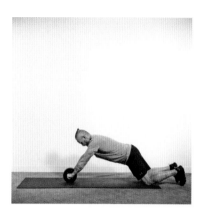

Kneel on the ground, holding the roller in front of you with both hands. Roll yourself out until you're engaging your core, hold for two seconds and then return to the start position. For diversity, you could be more adventurous and use a mix of angles: aim the roller to the left, to the right and then straight on.

EXERCISE 4: SIDE OBLIQUES BEND

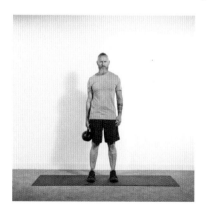 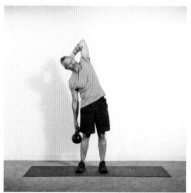 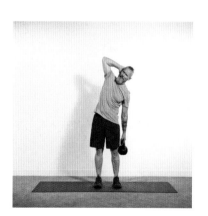

Stand with your feet shoulder-width apart, holding your chosen weight – which could be a kettlebell, plate or dumbbell – in one hand with a straight arm, and place your other hand on top of your head. Allow your body to lower to one side with the weight until you feel as though your core, abdominals and obliques are engaged, and your resistance item is below knee level. Return to the start position and repeat on the other side.

EXERCISE 5: OPPOSITE ELBOW TO KNEE CRUNCH

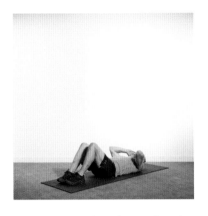 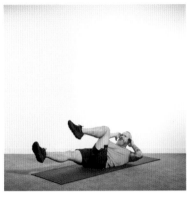 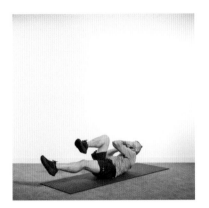

Lie on your back with your hands on your temples. Raise your left knee and bring your right elbow to meet it. Return to the start position. Now do the same with the other elbow and other knee.

FEEL AS THOUGH YOU'RE BEGINNING TO BREAK OLD HABITS, WHICH THEN ALLOWS YOU TO CREATE NEW ONES.

FULL BODY

Exercise 1: Your weakest legs exercise
Exercise 2: Push-up (see page 34)
Exercise 3: Band matrix (see page 31)
Exercise 4: Barbell row (see page 41)
Exercise 5: Clean and press (see page 41)

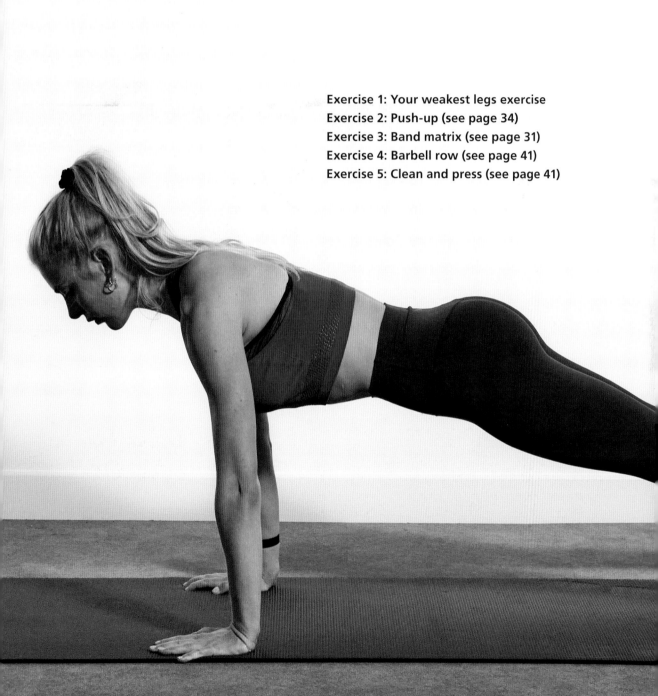

WEEK 1 RECAP

NUTRITION

○ Develop the habit of drinking water as soon as you get up in the morning.

○ Start to limit white, refined sugar. That stops your blood-sugar levels from fluctuating. This is important to avoid having sugar highs and sugar lows, which is when your energy levels spike and then crash.

○ Be conscious of your refined carbs intake. Refined means highly processed, such as white bread, white rice or white pasta. That will help you to keep track of how many calories you are having, should you want to bring that number down.

○ This is a good time to experiment and try new foods. That gives you diversity and also makes your digestive tract more efficient.

WELLBEING

○ Make your sleep a priority. You need to shut yourself down mentally and physically if you're to reboot and repair.

○ Why not try drinking a 'sleepy' tea before you go to bed? The process of making that drink will send a signal to the body that it's almost time for sleep.

○ In an ideal world, you won't be looking at your phone, or stimulating your brain, for at least an hour before bed.

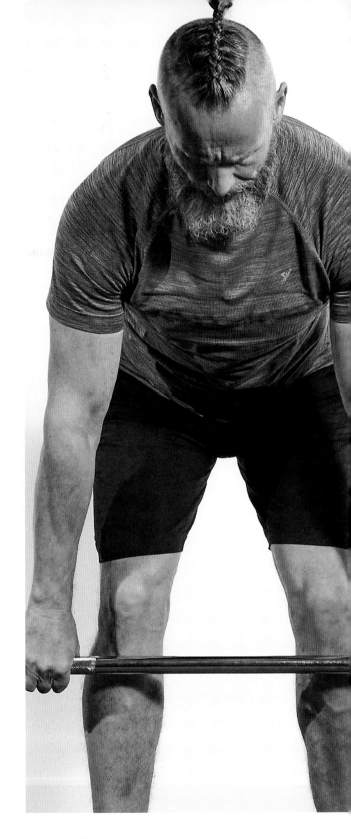

ACCUMULATOR: 5–2

LEGS MONDAY	1: Squat 2: Band matrix 3: Lunge 4: Box step 5: Hip thrust
UPPER-BODY TUESDAY	1: Push-up 2: Shoulder matrix 3: Arms matrix 4: Barbell row 5: Clean and press
DYNAMICS WEDNESDAY	1: Bear crawl into pigeon 2: Bear crawl into cobra 3: Sit-up with lumbar twist 4: Side crab 5: Plyometric with a jump
CORE THURSDAY	1: Plank to pike to shoulder taps 2: Crunches, leg raises and heel taps 3: Abdominal rollout with a roller 4: Side obliques bend 5: Opposite elbow to knee crunch
FULL-BODY FRIDAY	1: Your weakest legs exercise 2: Push-up 3: Band matrix 4: Barbell row 5: Clean and press
ACTIVE SATURDAY	Get out there and do all the things you wouldn't usually do, which will help you to feel free and alive. Why not do a mini-biathlon with a run and a bike ride?

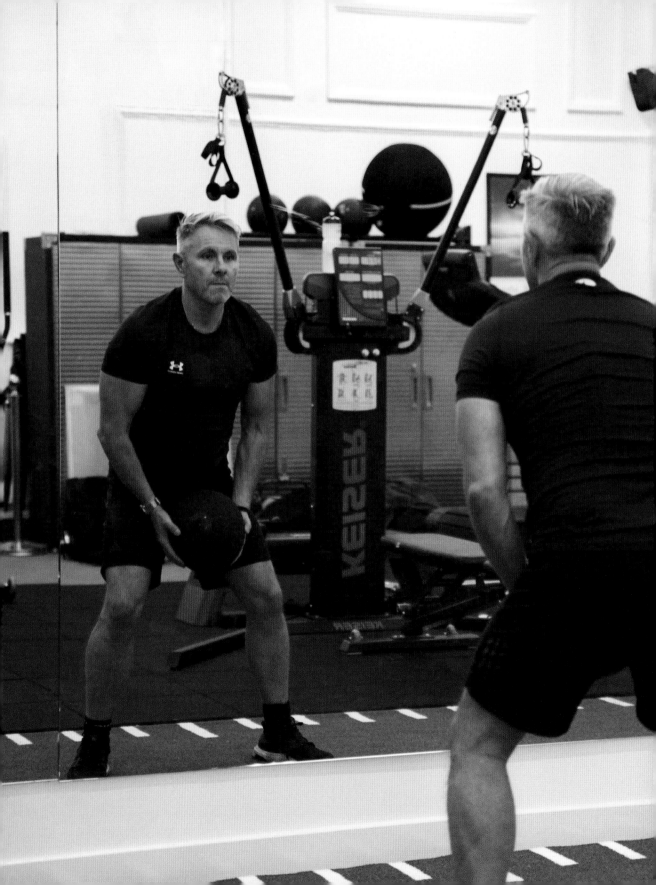

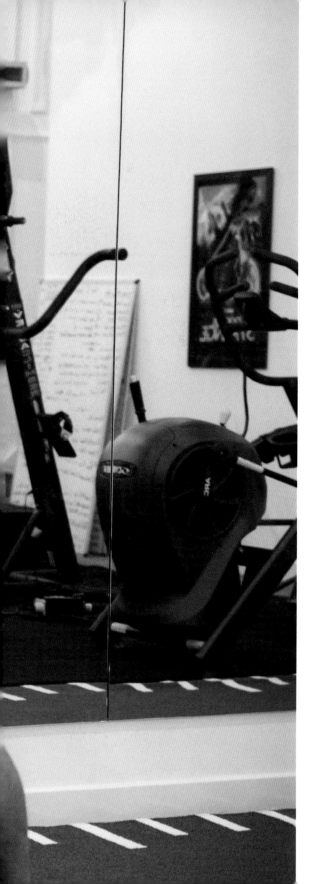

WEEK 2

'SIMON HAS A HOLISTIC APPROACH TO BODY CONDITIONING FOR ACTORS THAT IS SECOND TO NONE. IT'S A GREAT AND HIGHLY REWARDING PROGRAMME TO BE ON.'

Benedict Cumberbatch

FEELING IT

We all know that our mood can really affect what we feel we can achieve on any given day. We're dealing with our emotions all the time – sometimes tiredness and hormones, too. But if you can learn how to manage your mood, you can always get into the right mindset to progress your fitness.

ACCUMULATOR: 5–2

Part of an athlete's training is learning how to self-manage. Helped by visualization techniques and knowing where the finishing line is and which path to take to get there, they understand when to push and when to back off, while maintaining their fitness the majority of the time. That allows them to progress. If you're to get the most out of this challenge, you must try to do the same. When you feel as though you're able to push, that will accelerate your progression. But equally don't be afraid to sometimes ease off a little bit and adopt a 'less is more' mentality. You don't have to break records every day.

If you can develop your mental strength and stamina, the physicality tends to fall into place. For some, it might be the other way around, as working

out will help them mentally. But in my experience, it helps to be in the right headspace at the start of a challenge like this, because that allows you to get through any tough moments when you're not feeling your best. If you're doing a fitness programme for the first time, it's even more crucial that you're working on your mindset early on.

BEING IN THE PRESENT

Everyone's different, but you might find it helpful to get into the habit of doing a Monday morning mental wellbeing check-in (of course, you could do this every day if you like). It's a chance to be reflective, to be in the present and to feel how you're breathing and functioning. Do you feel alive and energized today or are you not fully in the present? We might find ourselves thinking about what we didn't do and what we need to do rather than concentrating on the here and now, and while you'll have a goal for this challenge, you shouldn't be looking too far into the future. The check-in is something you can do in the gym or at home before a workout, perhaps setting the alarm ten minutes early in order to run through it in bed before starting your day. Tailor it to whatever works for you and what will help you to self-regulate and maintain your mental wellbeing.

Here are a few questions you could ask yourself:

- How is my breathing?
- How is my heart rate?
- How are my concentration levels?
- How am I sleeping?
- How is my nutrition?
- How is my recovery?
- How motivated am I feeling today?
- What score would I give myself, between one and ten, for my mental and physical state?

While I would never insist that my clients do a regular mental health check-in, it's something I always speak to them about and would actively encourage if they thought it might help them. We know that the brain is a muscle, and so should be treated like any other muscle – you have to develop it and it's important to understand it. Sometimes

WEEK 2 KIT LIST

**ANKLE WEIGHTS
BANDS
BAR AND WEIGHTS
BENCH
BOX
DUMBBELLS
KETTLEBELL, PLATE
OR DUMBBELLS
ROLLER**

it's going to be sore and other times it's going to be super-efficient. What's important is how you deal with those moments in terms of developing effective ways of getting out of a sticky mental patch. Checking in with yourself and putting yourself in a more focused state should help to rectify that and keep you on track.

COMBATING ANXIETY

Focusing on your breathing, visualization and meditation are three very effective ways to deal with any feelings of anxiety and stress. It's interesting to

ARE YOU FEELING ALIVE AND ENERGIZED? CHECK IN WITH YOURSELF EVERY MONDAY MORNING.

understand that nasal breathing (breathing through your nose) is far better for you than breathing through your mouth. It seems more logical that you will get more oxygen and therefore more benefit from breathing in through your mouth, simply because it's bigger than the aperture of your nostrils. But the mouth has primarily been designed for eating and communicating, and the fact is that there are many more benefits of taking air through your nose. If you breathe in through your nose, you will get the right amount of oxygen and it will be the correct temperature, as your nose warms the air to body temperature, making it easier for your lungs to use. Air through your nose will also be distributed better through your body, as your nose releases nitric oxide, which helps to widen your blood vessels and therefore improves your circulation. Breathing in deeply through your nose has been shown to help reduce anxiety levels, and there are lots of exercises you can find online to explore this more.

Visualization is about identifying something you want, perceiving it and believing you can achieve it. This process can help you to complete a task, but also – and this might surprise you – it is thought to assist with repairing physical injuries. Research has shown the positive outcomes of visualization in athletes – by concentrating on an area of your body that you would like to repair and creating an image in your mind of the healing, your brain will send a signal, directing the right chemicals and helping the repair process to begin.

I also encourage my clients to meditate as it's great for enhancing your mental wellbeing and focusing your mind. If you're not already doing it, perhaps that's something you might want to explore this week.

FEELINGS RATHER THAN VISUALS

Get the mental side right and you'll be giving yourself the best possible foundation for the remaining weeks. If you're able to put in a strong first couple of weeks, you'll be starting to feel the changes in your body and mind. You're going to have to wait a little longer for those visible physical changes this week, but it's about feelings rather than visuals right now.

You might not have burned 5 pounds or 2 kilograms of fat from around your stomach (known as subcutaneous fat), but there's a chance you've burned that amount of fat from around your organs (called visceral fat), which is incredibly important. Your body tends to prioritize getting rid of fat from around your heart and lungs, creating space and releasing pressure on those organs, making your cardiovascular system more efficient. Maybe in Weeks 3 and 4, when all that is developing internally, the body will switch its priority and start burning the subcutaneous fat which will give you a visual reward. You'll be able to see that your body composition is changing. But for now, we need to be patient as we're laying the foundations for those changes.

'WITHOUT SIMON, I WOULDN'T HAVE MADE IT THROUGH FIFTEEN YEARS OF PLAYING BOND.'
Daniel Craig

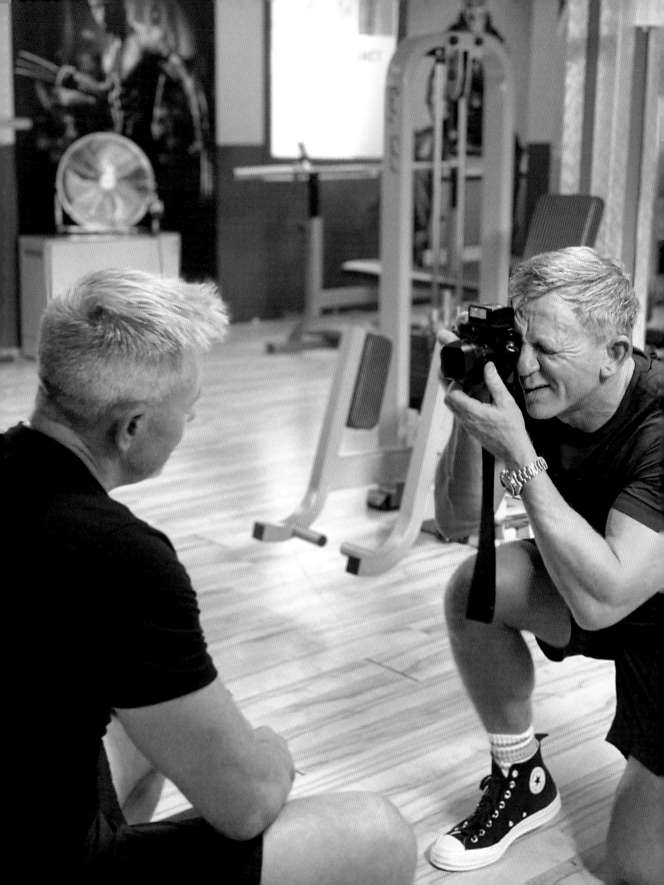

LEGS

EXERCISE 1: NARROW TO WIDE SQUAT

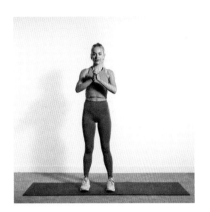

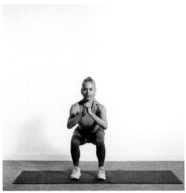

You're changing the angles from the regular squat in Week 1 – you're now switching from a narrow squat to a wide squat. For the narrow squat, your feet are pointing forwards rather than slightly outwards. Lower yourself down until your knees are at 90 degrees and hold that position for a count of four. Push up through your heels to return to the start position.

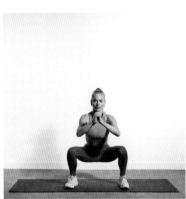

Now transition into the wide squat, with your feet further apart and pointing slightly outwards. Lower yourself down until your knees are at 90 degrees and hold that position for a count of four. Push up through your heels to return to the start position.

EXERCISE 2: BAND MATRIX WITH EXTRA SIDE SKIPS

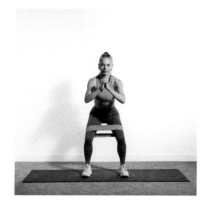 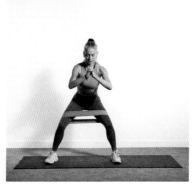 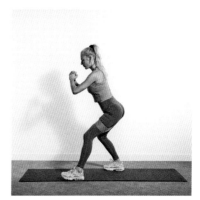

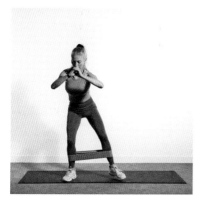 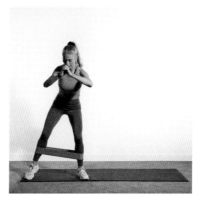

With a band just above your knees, position your feet so they are shoulder-width apart and then bend your knees slightly. Clasp your hands together in front of you while focusing straight ahead. Start with sidesteps, repeating small squat steps to the right and left, the number of reps dependent on what level you're exercising at. Maintaining tension in the band, put your left foot forward around 10 inches or 25 centimetres, and then move your right foot forward the same distance, before moving your left foot back followed by your right.

For the side skips, keep your knees locked and a neutral back. Placing the band halfway between your knees and your ankles, and maintaining its tension, do the required number of skip-jumps to the left and then the same number to the right to return back to the start position.

EXERCISE 3: LUNGE WITH RESISTANCE

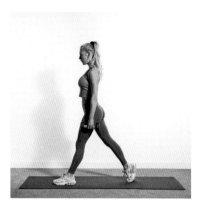 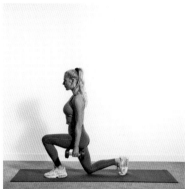

Stand with your feet shoulder-width apart, holding a kettlebell or two dumbbells. Lunge forward, dropping your rear leg until your knee kisses the floor. Explode upwards, returning to the start position. Swap the legs over, doing the same number of reps on each side.

YOU'RE INTO THE CHALLENGE NOW AND YOU'RE FEELING IT.

EXERCISE 4: BOX STEP WITH RESISTANCE AND KNEE DRIVE

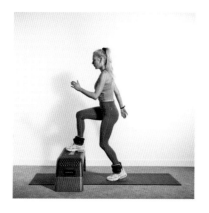 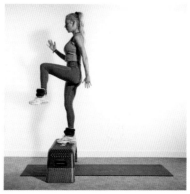 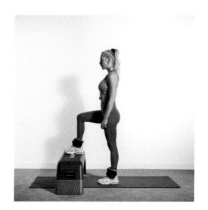

Wearing ankle weights, stand 10 inches or 25 centimetres back from the box with your feet shoulder-width apart and your arms by your sides. Step onto the box and in one continuous movement transition into a knee drive: you're lifting one knee off the ground so you're on one leg. Pause then lower the leg. Step down from the box. Do the reps and then swap legs.

EXERCISE 5: HIP THRUST WITH RESISTANCE

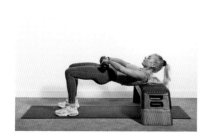 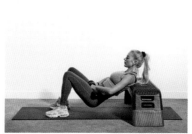

Holding a dumbbell in each hand, lie back, with your shoulder blades on the bench, your knees at 90 degrees and your feet shoulder-width apart. Resting the dumbbells on your hip bones, lower your glutes until they're about an inch or 2.5 centimetres off the ground. With control, return to the start position while contracting the glutes.

UPPER BODY

EXERCISE 1: PUSH-UP WITH DUMBBELLS WITH A MIX OF HAND POSITIONS

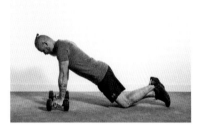
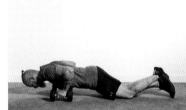
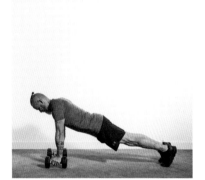
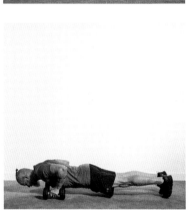

Variety is key for adaptation. For a mix of hand positions, adjust where the dumbbells are in relation to your shoulders. They can be shoulder-width apart, a little narrower or a little wider. Lower yourself down until your elbows are at 90 degrees. Push up and return to the start position, breathing out on exertion.

If you're a beginner, start with your knees on the ground. If you're at intermediate or advanced level, for extra intensity, take your knees off the ground and straighten your legs, keep a neutral back and neck, and do the same movement. You can freestyle this, doing different numbers of reps for each position, just so long as you get to the desired total. You might choose to do more reps of the position you find the easiest or you might want to challenge yourself by doing more of the position which you find the hardest.

EXERCISE 2: SHOULDER MATRIX WITH HALF MOVEMENTS

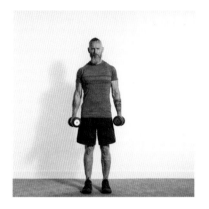 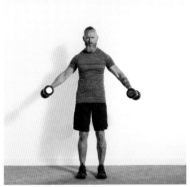

You're doing half movements for the lateral raises which means the muscles are under constant tension. For the lateral raises, lift the dumbbells to the side with slightly bent elbows so they are halfway to being level with your shoulders.

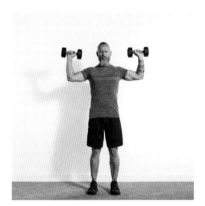 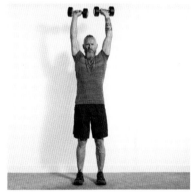

Return to the start position and transition from lateral raises into a shoulder press. Hold the dumbbells so that your arms are at 90 degrees on either side and the dumbbells are about 6 inches or 15 centimetres away from your ears. Raise the dumbbells into the air and then bring them together so they gently kiss. Bring them back down so your elbows and arms are at 90 degrees once again.

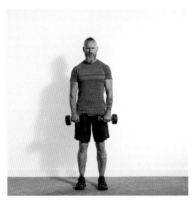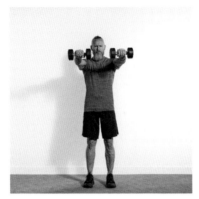

Transition into forward double raises. Hold the dumbbells so they are touching your thighs and then lift them up with a slightly bent elbow to shoulder height and return to the start position.

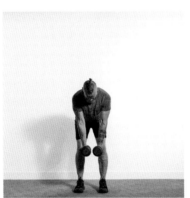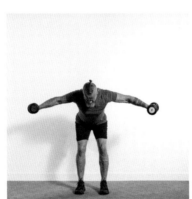

Transition into a bent-over row. Have a little bend in your knees. Maintain a neutral spine, back and neck. The dumbbells are dangling in front of you beneath your chest by your knees. With a slight bend in your elbows, retract the dumbbells so they are parallel with your shoulders, with a small contraction in your rear shoulders, and then return to the start position.

EXERCISE 3: ARMS MATRIX (SEE PAGE 38)

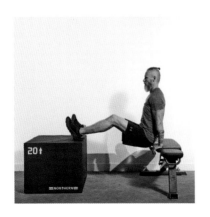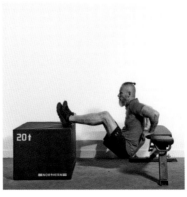

For added resistance when doing tricep dips, use two benches, so that your legs are raised. Lower yourself down until your elbows are at 90 degrees. Return to start position.

EXERCISE 4: BARBELL ROW PLYOMETRIC

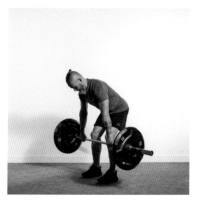
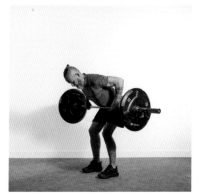

After adding the right amount of weights to suit your ability, place the barbell in front of you. Bend your knees. Keeping a neutral back, use an overhand grip to clasp the barbell and bring it up to your knees. Slide the bar up your thighs into your waist, retracting the back and squeezing the lats.

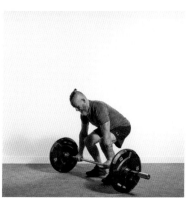
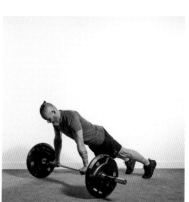

Put the barbell down on the ground. To start the plyometric movement, shoot your legs back and then jump your feet back towards the bar. Get back into the original position and repeat.

EXERCISE 5: CLEAN AND PRESS (SEE PAGE 41)

DYNAMIC STRETCHING

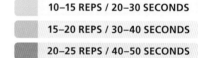

10–15 REPS / 20–30 SECONDS
15–20 REPS / 30–40 SECONDS
20–25 REPS / 40–50 SECONDS

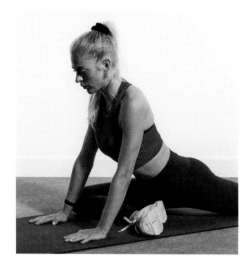

Exercise 1: Bear crawl into pigeon (see page 42)

Exercise 2: Bear crawl into cobra (see page 43)

Exercise 3: Sit-up with lumbar twist (see page 43)

Exercise 4: Side crab (see page 44)

Exercise 5: Plyometric with a jump (see page 45)

WEEK 2 / **THURSDAY**

CORE

10–15 REPS / 20–30 SECONDS
15–20 REPS / 30–40 SECONDS
20–25 REPS / 40–50 SECONDS

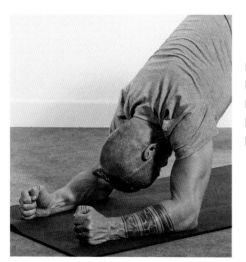

Exercise 1: Plank to pike to shoulder taps (see page 47)

Exercise 2: Crunches, leg raises and heel taps (see page 48)

Exercise 3: Abdominal rollout with a roller (see page 49)

Exercise 4: Side obliques bend (see page 49)

Exercise 5: Opposite elbow to knee crunch (see page 50)

FULL BODY

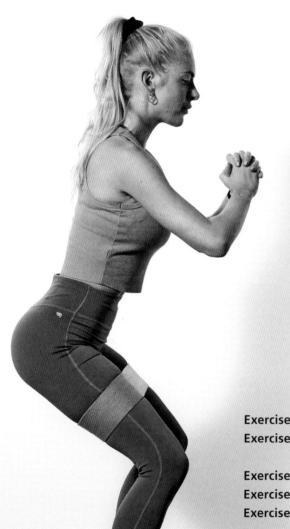

Exercise 1: Your weakest legs exercise

Exercise 2: Push-up with dumbbells with a mix of hand positions (see page 64)

Exercise 3: Band matrix with extra side skips (see page 61)

Exercise 4: Barbell row plyometric (see page 67)

Exercise 5: Clean and press (see page 41)

WEEK 2 RECAP

NUTRITION

○ Eat a 'rainbow' diet, with as many colours on your plate as possible, as that will help to give you diversity and encourage you to choose foods that are high in nutrients.

○ If you usually have cow's milk, why not try a nut milk and see how it goes? It can be a good source of vitamins and when unsweetened, lower in calories too.

○ Be preventative. If you know you always have a craving at 3 or 4 p.m., have a glass of water and a healthy snack half an hour before. Create a habit that's going to be sustainable for this challenge and beyond.

WELLBEING

○ Avoid tea, coffee and sugary drinks before going to bed as they will disturb your sleep.

○ The body loves a routine, so having the same bedtime each night will help you to get good quality sleep.

○ If you're training in the evening, try to ensure that you finish your workout at least two hours before you go to bed, as that will give your body time to stabilize and relax.

○ Make your workout as convenient as possible, which means training as close to home as you can, because that reduces the chance of you finding an excuse to miss a session this week.

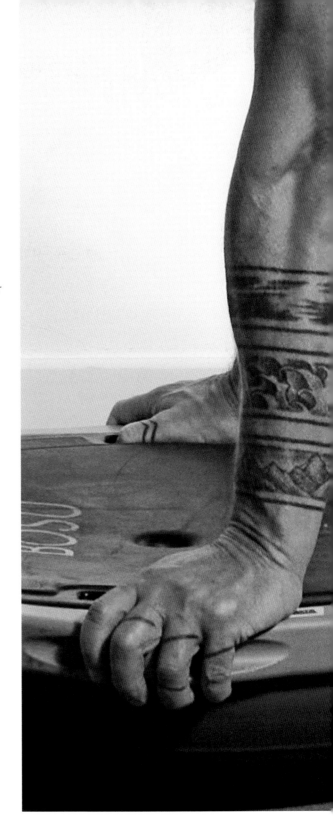

ACCUMULATOR: 5–2

LEGS MONDAY	1: Narrow to wide squat 2: Band matrix with extra side skips 3: Lunge with resistance 4: Box step with resistance and knee drive 5: Hip thrust with resistance
UPPER-BODY TUESDAY	1: Push-up with dumbbells with a mix of hand positions 2: Shoulder matrix with half movements 3: Arms matrix 4: Barbell row plyometric 5: Clean and press
DYNAMICS WEDNESDAY	1: Bear crawl into pigeon 2: Bear crawl into cobra 3: Sit-up with lumbar twist 4: Side crab 5: Plyometric with a jump
CORE THURSDAY	1: Plank to pike to shoulder taps 2: Crunches, leg raises and heel taps 3: Abdominal rollout with a roller 4: Side obliques bend 5: Opposite elbow to knee crunch
FULL-BODY FRIDAY	1: Your weakest legs exercise 2: Push-up with dumbbells 3: Band matrix with extra side skips 4: Barbell row plyometric 5: Clean and press
ACTIVE SATURDAY	Why not ride your bike today? When was the last time you went for a long cycle ride?

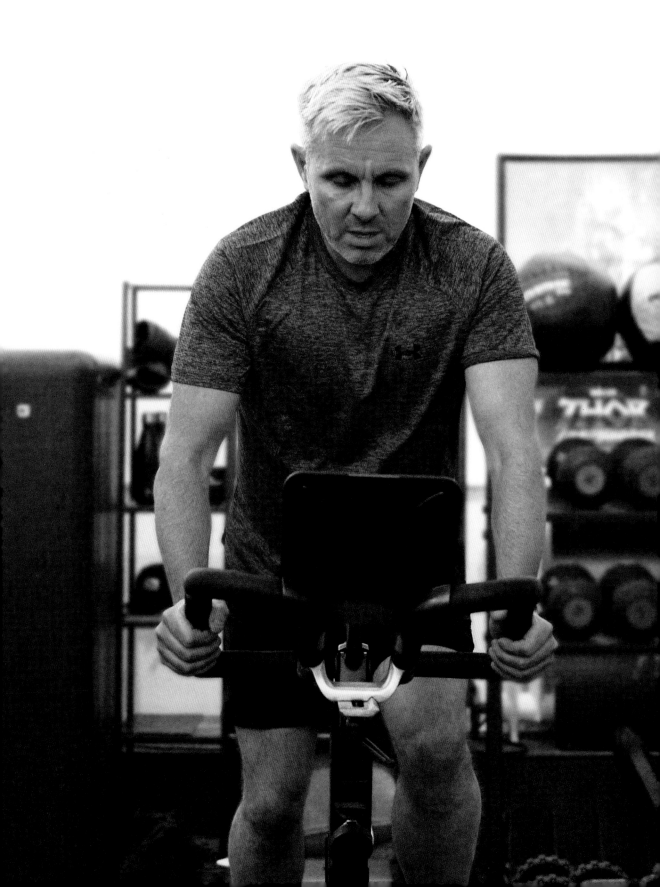

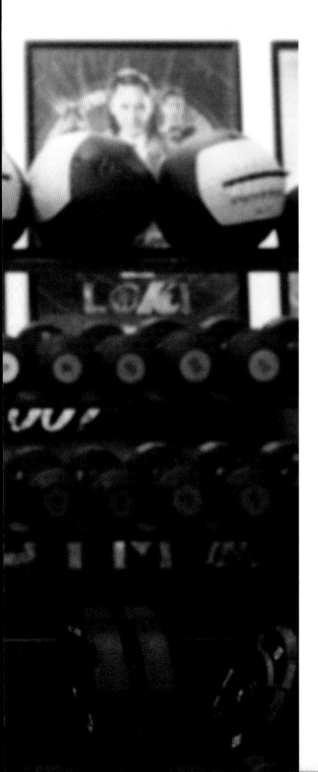

WEEK 3

'SIMON IS A
NO-NONSENSE
TRAINER – WITHOUT
PRETENSION. HE
HAS AN INCREDIBLE
WEALTH OF
EXPERIENCE.'
Rachel Weisz

MAKING PROGRESS

The more efficient and fitter your body becomes, the more you need specific nutrition for energy, repair and detoxing. Your nutrition needs to be balanced and relevant to what you're doing and hoping to achieve.

ACCUMULATOR: 5–2

With each week of this challenge, your nutrition becomes increasingly important. In the first couple of weeks, you could have taken the first few steps, such as eliminating most sugary snacks from your kitchen cupboards. Now, in Week 3, when you should be starting to feel as though you're making progress with the challenge, you should be refining what you're putting in your supermarket trolley or choosing for an online shop. Your body is going to tell you that tailoring your nutrition is now a necessity. Try to listen to what it's saying.

Be aware of what you're eating for repair and energy, and also how you will get the good essential fats and fatty acids that will help to maintain good hormonal levels (think avocados, nuts and some fish). You're ditching old habits and creating new ones, always tailoring and refining your own take on nutrition to support what you're doing physically.

WORK IN PROGRESS

It helps to think of your nutrition as a work in progress that will always be changing. While your calorie intake might stay the same, you could change your 'macros' – the percentage of your calories that come from proteins, carbohydrates and good fats – from week to week. Your take on nutrition will naturally depend on what your goals are for this ten-week challenge. If you're looking to lose some weight, for example, you'll need to be in a calorie deficit, which is when your output is exceeding your input and you're using more calories than you're consuming.

You might decide to split each of your three meals a day in half and eat six 'brunches' a day. Or you might prefer three main meals and snacks. Or perhaps you could opt for intermittent fasting where you only eat in a six-hour window during the day, with one big meal at the beginning and another at the end of that window, giving you an eighteen-hour fast. For instance, you could eat a meal at 9 a.m. and another at 3 p.m. and then you wouldn't eat again until 9 a.m. the following morning. How you use food depends on the results you want and what's sustainable for you. And I always believe that nothing is off the table. If you tell yourself that you're not allowed something, your focus will be affected detrimentally because you'll find you'll become obsessed with what you can't have. Psychologically, it's far better to tell yourself that you can eat what you want, in moderation.

A MORE SUSTAINABLE APPROACH

Allow yourself an occasional beer or glass of wine this week if you fancy it. When people are doing a fitness challenge, they tend to moderate how much they are drinking. Maybe you will want to have a glass of something on a Friday or Saturday night to celebrate getting through the week. And

that's absolutely fine, and also a more sustainable approach than completely cutting out alcohol. We're all social creatures and you might want to have a drink with friends or family to help you to decompress. If you usually enjoy a drink, and then you don't have one for ten weeks, you're likely to make up for it after you have completed the challenge. But don't see alcohol as a reward for completing this programme: your reward should be your health. Remember that this challenge isn't just about these ten weeks, but also about learning new habits for the rest of your life.

WEEK 3 KIT LIST

BAND
BAR WITH WEIGHTS
BENCHES
BOSU
BOX
DUMBBELLS
KETTLEBELL, PLATE
OR DUMBBELLS
ROLLER

YOUR MUSCLES AREN'T MADE IN THE GYM – THEY'RE MADE IN THE KITCHEN.

LEGS

	10–15 REPS / 20–30 SECONDS
	15–20 REPS / 30–40 SECONDS
	20–25 REPS / 40–50 SECONDS

EXERCISE 1: BOSU SQUAT

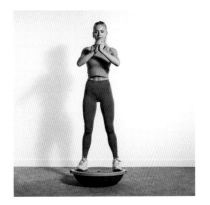 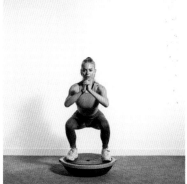

Stand on a BOSU, hard side up, which adds some instability, with your feet shoulder-width apart and your toes pointing slightly outwards. Lower yourself down until your knees are at 90 degrees and hold that position for a count of four. Push up through your heels to return to the start position.

NOTHING'S OFF THE TABLE – IF YOU TELL YOURSELF YOU CAN'T HAVE SOMETHING, YOU'LL ONLY OBSESS OVER IT.

EXERCISE 2: BAND MATRIX WITH A SECOND BAND

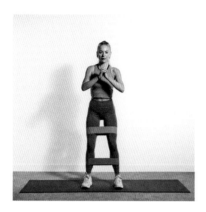 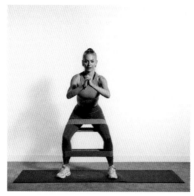 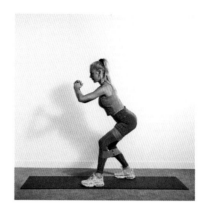

With the first band just above your knees and the second band just above your ankles, position your feet so they are shoulder-width apart and bend your knees slightly. Clasp your hands together in front of you while focusing straight ahead. Start with sidesteps, doing squat shuffles to the right and then to the left, the number of reps dependent on which level you're exercising at.

Now put your left foot forward around 10 inches or 25 centimetres until you get tension on the band, and then move your right foot forward the same distance, before moving your left foot back and then your right.

EXERCISE 3: SPRINTER LUNGE ON THE BOSU WITH KNEE DRIVE

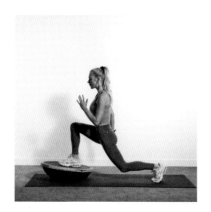 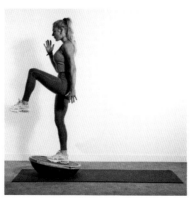

With the BOSU hard side up, put one foot in the middle while keeping the other leg behind you in a lunge position. Bring the rear leg forward so you're standing, and then raise the knee of the same leg to 90 degrees so you're standing on one leg. Return to the start position. Change to the other leg and repeat.

EXERCISE 4: BOX JUMP

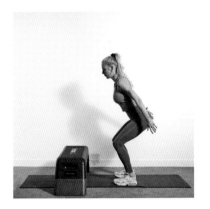 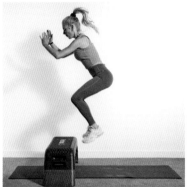

Stand 10 inches or 25 centimetres back from the box with your feet shoulder-width apart and your arms by your sides. Get into a squat position. Propel yourself through the air. Land with both feet on the box in a squat position and extend your legs to a standing position. Step down from the box and return to the start position.

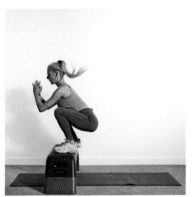 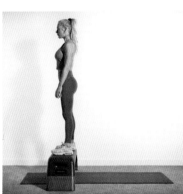

EXERCISE 5: ONE-LEGGED HIP THRUST

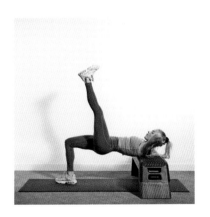 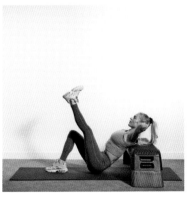

Lie back, with your shoulder blades on the bench, and extend one leg straight up in the air. Lower your glutes until they're about an inch or 2.5 centimetres off the ground. Return to the start position while contracting the glutes, and then repeat with the other leg.

UPPER BODY

▨	10–15 REPS / 20–30 SECONDS
▨	15–20 REPS / 30–40 SECONDS
▨	20–25 REPS / 40–50 SECONDS

EXERCISE 1: PUSH-UP ON A BOSU

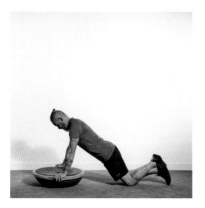
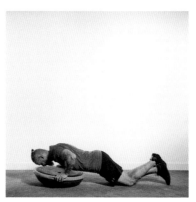

Place your hands on each side of the BOSU (hard side up). If this exercise is fairly new to you, you might find it easier to start with your knees on the ground with your ankles crossed behind you. Lower yourself down until your elbows are at 90 degrees. Push up and return to the start position, breathing out on exertion.

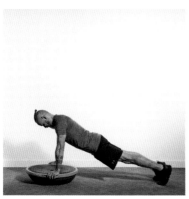
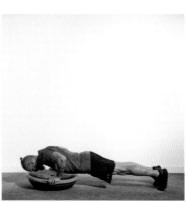

For extra intensity, take your knees off the ground and straighten your legs, keep a neutral back and neck, and do the same movement.

EXERCISE 2: SHOULDER MATRIX SEATED

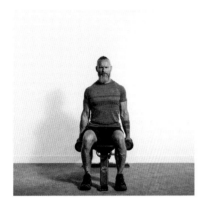 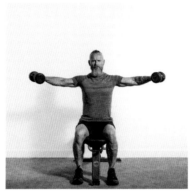

You're sitting down, which means you can't use your legs and you're isolating the upper body. For the lateral raises, lift the dumbbells to the side with slightly bent elbows so they are level with your shoulders. Return to the start position.

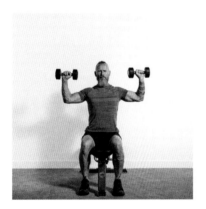 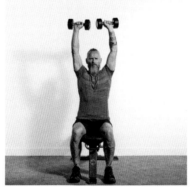

Transition from lateral raises into a shoulder press. Hold the dumbbells so that your arms are at 90 degrees on either side and the dumbbells are about 6 inches or 15 centimetres away from your ears. Raise the dumbbells into the air and then bring them together so they gently kiss. Bring them back down so your elbows and arms are at 90 degrees and repeat.

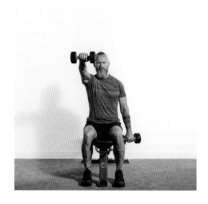 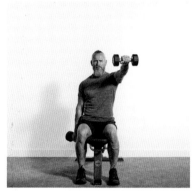

Transition into forward raises. Hold the dumbbells so they are touching your thighs and then lift one dumbbell up with a slightly bent elbow to shoulder height and return to the start position. Repeat on the other side.

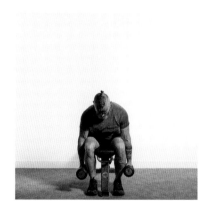 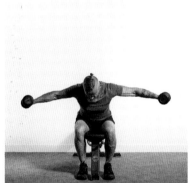

Transition into a bent-over row. Maintain a neutral spine, back and neck. The dumbbells are dangling in front of you beneath your chest and by your shins. With a slight bend in your elbows, retract the dumbbells so they are level with your shoulders and then return to the start position.

EXERCISE 3: ARMS MATRIX SEATED

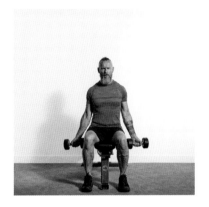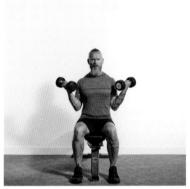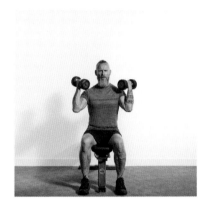

You're sitting down on a bench, which isolates the muscles. Hold a dumbbell in each hand so they are about 6 inches or 15 centimetres away from your legs, with your palms facing away from your body. Slowly raise your dumbbells up to shoulder height. Lift your elbows a couple of inches or 5 centimetres higher for extra pressure and then return to the start position.

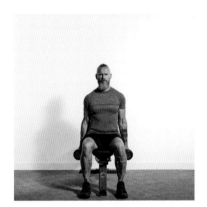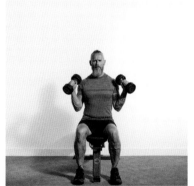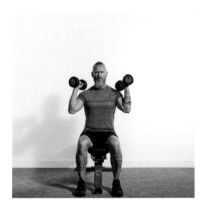

Change the hand position so your palms are now facing your body and the dumbbells are close to your legs. Curl the dumbbells up to shoulder height and then, with a little tip of the elbows which applies extra pressure on the bicep, return to the start position.

You'll need a bench for triceps dips. For added resistance, use two benches and raise your legs (see pages 39 and 66). You should almost be sitting on your hands, with your fingers coming off the edge of the bench. Lower yourself down until your elbows are at 90 degrees. Return to the start position.

EXERCISE 4: INCLINE DOUBLE DUMBBELLS

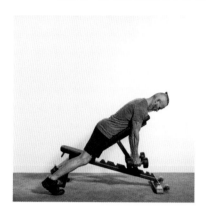 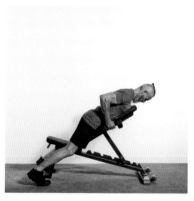

Lie on a bench on your front with a 45-degree incline, holding a moderate dumbbell in each hand in front of you. Retract the dumbbells together and squeeze your shoulder blades together until the dumbbells are level with your chest, and then return to the start position.

EXERCISE 5: CLEAN AND PRESS (SEE PAGE 41)

YOUR BODY WANTS TO DO EVERYTHING AT 100 PER CENT AND IN THE MOST EFFICIENT WAY. YOUR JOB IS TO FACILITATE THAT.

DYNAMIC STRETCHING

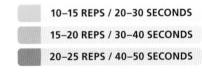	10–15 REPS / 20–30 SECONDS
	15–20 REPS / 30–40 SECONDS
	20–25 REPS / 40–50 SECONDS

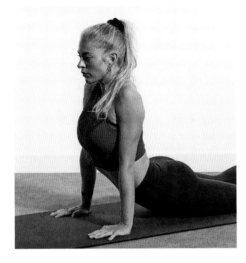

Exercise 1: Bear crawl into pigeon (see page 42)

Exercise 2: Bear crawl into cobra (see page 43)

Exercise 3: Sit-up with lumbar twist (see page 43)

Exercise 4: Side crab (see page 44)

Exercise 5: Plyometric with a jump (see page 45)

WEEK 3 / **THURSDAY**

CORE

	10–15 REPS / 20–30 SECONDS
	15–20 REPS / 30–40 SECONDS
	20–25 REPS / 40–50 SECONDS

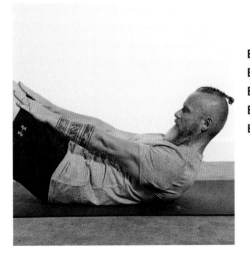

Exercise 1: Plank to pike to shoulder taps (see page 47)

Exercise 2: Crunches, leg raises and heel taps (see page 48)

Exercise 3: Abdominal rollout with a roller (see page 49)

Exercise 4: Side obliques bend (see page 49)

Exercise 5: Opposite elbow to knee crunch (see page 50)

FULL BODY

	10–15 REPS / 20–30 SECONDS
	15–20 REPS / 30–40 SECONDS
	20–25 REPS / 40–50 SECONDS

Exercise 1: Your weakest legs exercise
Exercise 2: Push-up on a BOSU (see page 79)
Exercise 3: Band matrix with a second band (see page 77)
Exercise 4: Incline double dumbbells (see page 83)
Exercise 5: Clean and press (see page 41)

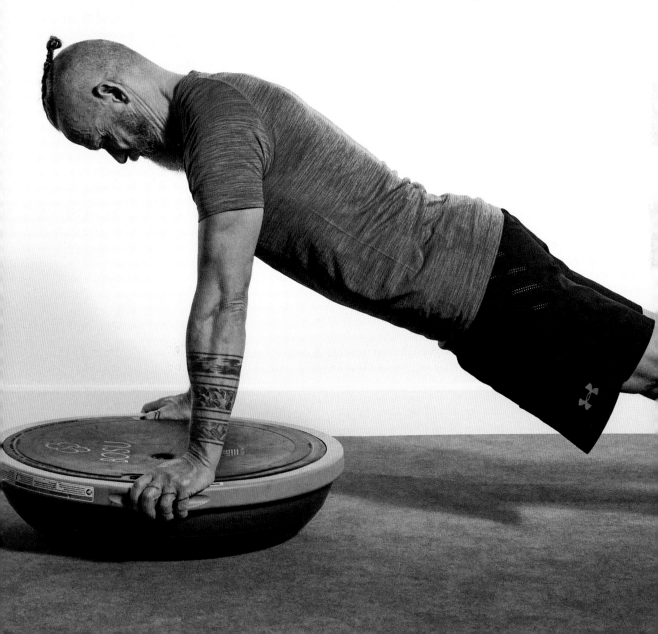

WEEK 3 RECAP

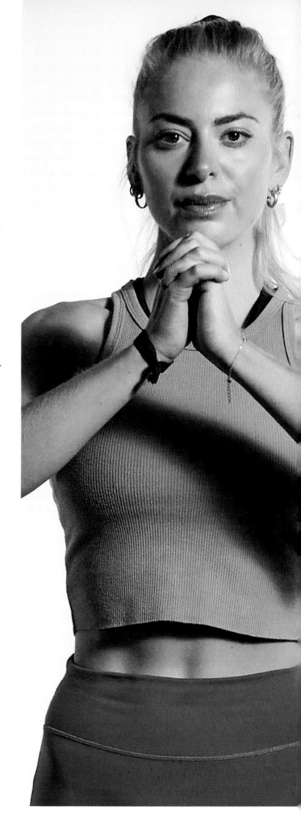

NUTRITION

○ Moving away from ultra-processed food and buying fresh, quality ingredients to cook with is a game-changer. We're all under time constraints, but avoiding processed food can have a huge effect on how you feel. You'll be consuming foods that are packed with the nutrients the body needs for energy and repair.

○ If you like coffee, why not have one half an hour before your workout, which is going to stimulate your brain and help transition you into activity mode.

○ Copy the Italians by having a glass of water with your espresso, ensuring you're hydrated as well as stimulated.

○ Try to consume something within thirty minutes of finishing training because that's when your body will be most receptive to certain food groups. Ideally, you need a blend of carbohydrates and protein, with the carbs giving you energy and the protein helping with repair.

WELLBEING

○ Understand that mental fatigue will stop you a long time before physical fatigue does. Look after yourself this week, and do those regular check-ins.

○ If you're struggling to sleep at the moment, could you stay with a friend for a couple of nights, or even try sleeping in a different room? Changing your environment can break the pattern of bad sleep.

○ Needless to say, worrying about bad sleep can be really counterproductive. Tell yourself you're capable of getting good-quality sleep, and if it doesn't happen tonight, it'll improve soon. You're in control.

ACCUMULATOR: 5–2

LEGS MONDAY	1: BOSU squat 2: Band matrix with a second band 3: Sprinter lunge on the BOSU with a knee drive 4: Box jump 5: One-legged hip thrust
UPPER-BODY TUESDAY	1: Push-up on a BOSU 2: Shoulder matrix seated 3: Arms matrix seated 4: Incline double dumbbells 5: Clean and press
DYNAMICS WEDNESDAY	1: Bear crawl into pigeon 2: Bear crawl into cobra 3: Sit-up with lumbar twist 4: Side crab 5: Plyometric with a jump
CORE THURSDAY	1: Plank to pike to shoulder taps 2: Crunches, leg raises and heel taps 3: Abdominal rollout with a roller 4: Side obliques bend 5: Opposite elbow to knee crunch
FULL-BODY FRIDAY	1: Your weakest legs exercise 2: Push-up on a BOSU 3: Band matrix with a second band 4: Incline double dumbbells 5: Clean and press
ACTIVE SATURDAY	Swimming, yoga, Pilates, running … Try to do an eclectic mix of activities from week to week.

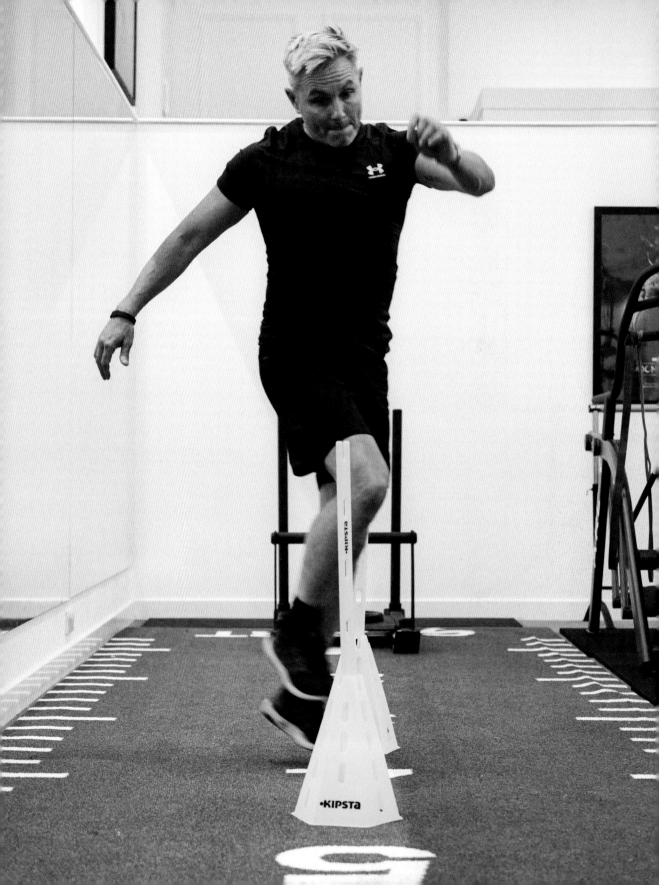

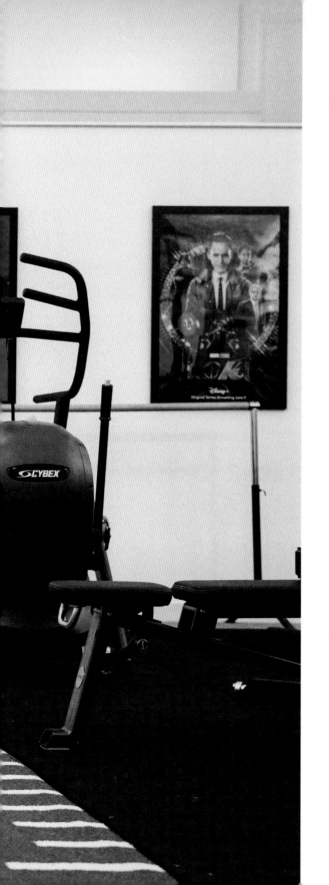

WEEK 4

'SIMON IS NOT ONLY ONE OF THE SMARTEST TRAINERS I'VE EVER MET, BUT HE'S ALSO ONE OF THE KINDEST HUMAN BEINGS.'
Dave Bautista

TIME TO PUSH

By now, your body should be used to the movement patterns in this programme. You're starting to see the fruits of your labour. You're beginning to feel as though you're making real progress. Perhaps things are getting easier. You're feeling committed and hopefully thinking: 'I'm enjoying this.'

ACCUMULATOR: 5–3

If you think that you're ready to do so, you might want to push a little harder now than you did in the first three weeks, but don't take that to the extreme.

At this stage, you should be more comfortable with this challenge. I'm hoping you've found a balance with your training, recovery and nutrition, or you're close to achieving that. You've integrated fitness into your lifestyle, which means everything feels more natural, and a lot easier than it was at the beginning. Maybe in the first three weeks of the challenge, you always had to think about what you were doing, which required a fair amount of mental energy, but now you're getting on with the exercises almost subconsciously. That's great, as it should take away some of the stresses and strains, and the

programme should be boosting your energy. This is now part of your daily routine, and you're already feeling the benefits.

As your body has steadily become capable of doing more, you might wish to make use of that new capability, perhaps even to progress on the reps from beginner to intermediate or from intermediate to advanced, and maybe also choose slightly heavier weights. But don't feel as though you have to, as you can also keep going at the same level. It's up to you.

JUST A MINUTE

One change you will notice this week is that I'm increasing your cardio between exercises from two minutes to three. You should be able to handle that extra minute now. If you had been planning on losing weight, perhaps you've burned a few pounds by now. I'm sure your lung capacity will have improved since Week 1 as your body should now be becoming generally more efficient. Your VO$_2$ Max – which is the maximum amount of oxygen your body can use during exercise – will have gone up. Significantly, your recovery rate will also be better. You should be capable of doing three minutes of cardio as your heart rate will quickly stabilize, allowing you to get back into the exercises again. At this stage of the challenge, your body should have built up its ability to deal with lactic acid and other toxins, which are produced after a workout. Flushing out those toxins will reduce the chances of delayed-onset muscle soreness. You're no longer working outside your comfort zone.

WORKING ON YOUR WEAKNESSES

If I'm training an actor for a film, I'll have a good idea of someone's capabilities by Week 4. I'll be assessing their strengths and weaknesses, seeing what they're capable of and evaluating which areas might need some additional focus and encouragement. You might want to do a similar personal analysis – ask yourself what you're good at and what you're finding most challenging. Be honest with yourself. You might even want to note down your strengths and weaknesses, perhaps picking out two or three exercises that you're enjoying the most as well as the same number of exercises that you find harder. Towards the end of the challenge, you could look back at what you have written and see how you have progressed. Do you still have the same weaknesses or is there another muscle group or movement that needs attention?

Working on your weaknesses will help you to enhance your strengths. There's a reason that the

WEEK 4 KIT LIST

BANDS
BARBELL
BENCHES
BOSU
BOX
DUMBBELLS (with option of a kettlebell or a medicine ball too)

full-body workout on a Friday always includes the legs exercise that you struggle with the most: it encourages you to think about which aspects of your training need improvement.

I'm introducing new dynamic stretching and core exercises this week (having had the same ones for the first three weeks).

LEGS

	10–15 REPS / 20–30 SECONDS
	15–20 REPS / 30–40 SECONDS
	20–25 REPS / 40–50 SECONDS

EXERCISE 1: BOSU GOBLET SQUAT

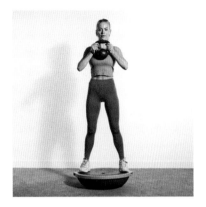 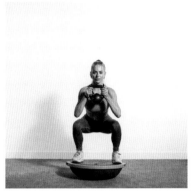

Holding dumbbells, a kettlebell or a medicine ball, stand on a BOSU hard side up, which adds some instability, with your feet shoulder-width apart and your toes pointing slightly outwards. Lower yourself down until your knees are at 90 degrees and hold that position for a count of four. Push up through your heels to return to the start position.

YOUR BODY IS BECOMING MORE EFFICIENT AND YOU CAN DO MORE, SO PUSH A LITTLE HARDER IF YOU CAN.

EXERCISE 2: BAND MATRIX WITH A SECOND BAND AND EXTRA SIDE SKIPS

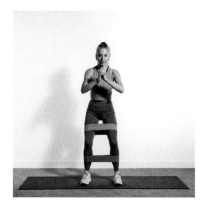 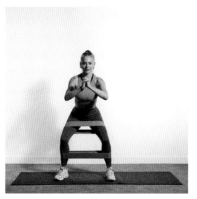 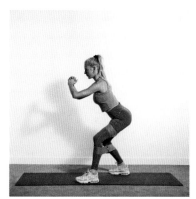

With the first band just above your knees and the second band just above your ankles, position your feet so they are shoulder-width apart and bend your legs slightly. Clasp your hands together in front of you while focusing straight ahead. Start with sidesteps, repeating small squat steps to the right and left, the number of reps dependent on what level you're exercising at. Then, maintaining tension in the band, put your left foot forward around 10 inches or 25 centimetres, and then move your right foot forward the same distance, before moving your left foot back followed by your right.

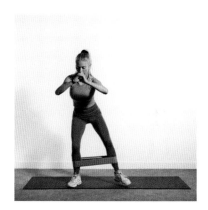 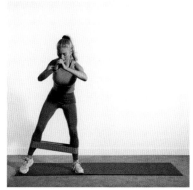

For the side skips, keep your knees locked and a neutral back. Now with just one band placed below your knee, maintain its tension, and skip-jump to the left. Once you've completed your reps on that side, do the same on the other side to return to the starting position.

EXERCISE 3: SPRINTER LUNGE ON THE BOSU WITH RESISTANCE

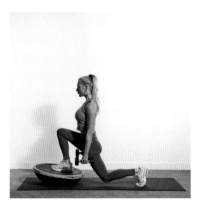 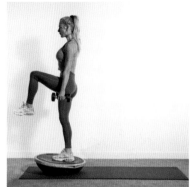

With the BOSU hard side up and holding a dumbbell in each hand, place one foot in the middle of the BOSU while keeping the other foot behind you in a lunge position. Bring the rear leg forward so you're standing on the BOSU, and then raise the knee of the same leg to 90 degrees so you're standing on one leg. Return to the start position. Change to the other leg and repeat.

EXERCISE 4: BOX JUMP WITH RESISTANCE

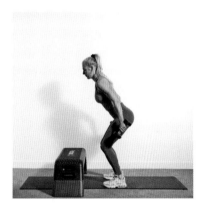 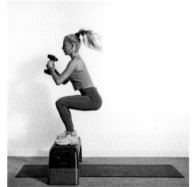

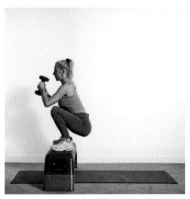 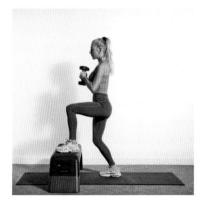

Holding a dumbbell in each hand, stand 10 inches or 25 centimetres back from the box with your feet shoulder-width apart and your arms by your sides. Get into a squat position. Propel yourself through the air and land with both feet on the box in a squat position. Now extend your legs to a standing position. Step down from the box and return to the start position.

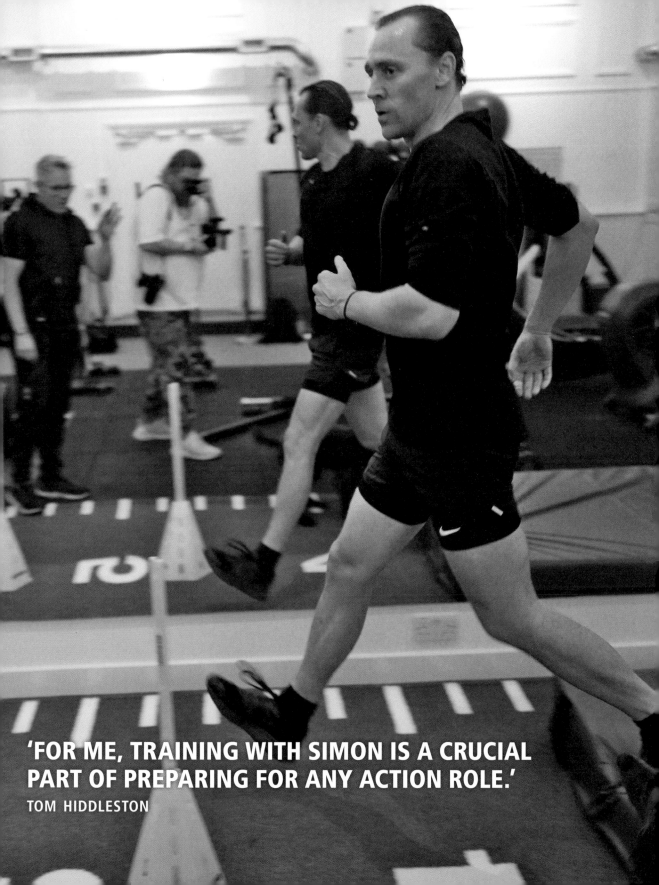

'FOR ME, TRAINING WITH SIMON IS A CRUCIAL PART OF PREPARING FOR ANY ACTION ROLE.'
TOM HIDDLESTON

EXERCISE 5: ONE-LEGGED HIP THRUST WITH RESISTANCE

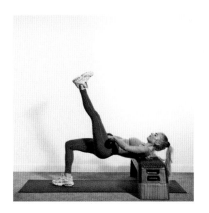 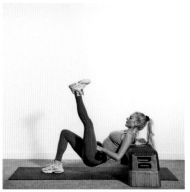

Lie back, holding a dumbbell in each hand, with your shoulder blades on the bench, one leg straight up in the air. Rest the dumbbells on your hip bones and lower your glutes until they're about an inch or 2.5 centimetres off the ground. Return to the start position while contracting the glutes.

YOU SHOULD NOW FEEL IN TUNE WITH THIS CHALLENGE AND HAVE ESTABLISHED A BALANCE WITH YOUR TRAINING, RECOVERY AND NUTRITION.

UPPER BODY

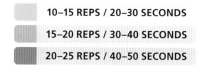

	10–15 REPS / 20–30 SECONDS
	15–20 REPS / 30–40 SECONDS
	20–25 REPS / 40–50 SECONDS

EXERCISE 1: PUSH-UP WITH A KNEE DRIVE

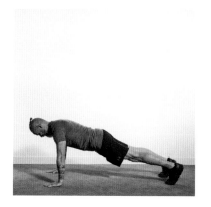
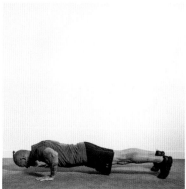

Place your hands on the ground, shoulder-width apart. Lower yourself down until your elbows are at 90 degrees. Push up and return to the start position, breathing out on exertion. Lift and drive one knee forward then the other, alternating between the legs.

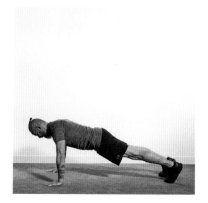
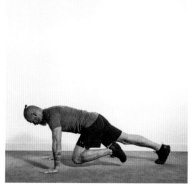

EXERCISE 2: SHOULDER MATRIX SEATED WITH HALF MOVEMENTS

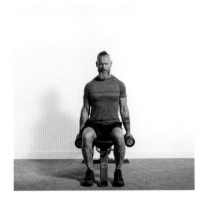 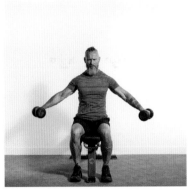

You're sitting down, which means you can't use your legs and you're isolating the upper body. You're doing half movements for the lateral raises, so the muscles are under constant tension. For the lateral raises, lift the dumbbells to the side with slightly bent elbows, so they are halfway to being level with your shoulders. Return to the start position.

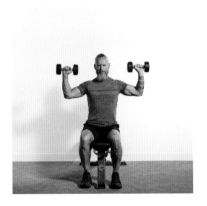 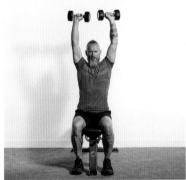

Transition from lateral raises into a shoulder press. Hold the dumbbells so that your arms are at 90 degrees on either side and the dumbbells are about 6 inches or 15 centimetres away from your ears. Raise the dumbbells into the air and then bring them together so they gently kiss. Bring them back down so your elbows and arms are at 90 degrees once again.

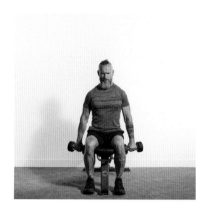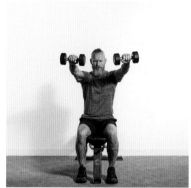

Transition into forward double raises. Hold the dumbbells so they are touching your thighs and then lift both dumbbells up with slightly bent elbows to shoulder height, and return to the start position.

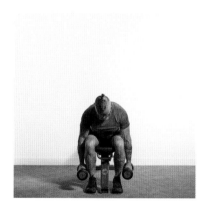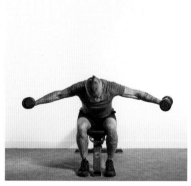

Transition into a bent-over row. Maintain a neutral spine, back and neck. The dumbbells are dangling down by your shins. With a slight bend in your elbows, retract the dumbbells so they are level with your shoulders and then return to the start position.

EXERCISE 3: ARMS MATRIX SEATED (SEE PAGE 82)

EXERCISE 4: INCLINE SINGLE-ARM DUMBBELLS

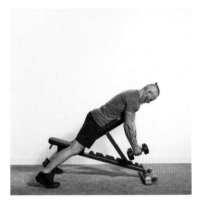 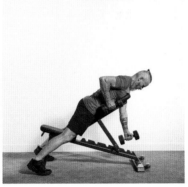

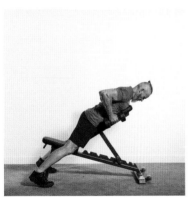 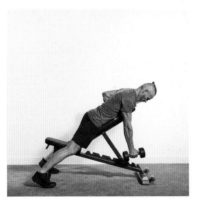

Lie on a bench with a 45-degree incline, holding a moderate dumbbell in front of you in each hand. Retract one dumbbell to your chest while keeping the other in front of you. Return to the start position and repeat with the other arm.

EXERCISE 5: CLEAN AND PRESS (SEE PAGE 41)

DYNAMIC STRETCHING

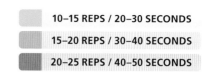

10–15 REPS / 20–30 SECONDS	
15–20 REPS / 30–40 SECONDS	
20–25 REPS / 40–50 SECONDS	

EXERCISE 1: LOWER LUMBAR STRETCH

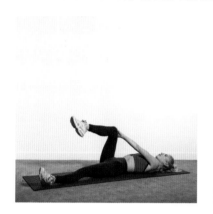
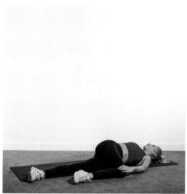

Lying on your back with your legs straight, bring your right leg over your left as far as you can. Extend your right arm across the floor to the right. Bring your left hand to your right leg, and apply pressure on your knee, lowering it towards the floor on your left. Turn your head in the opposite direction and focus on your fingers. Return to the start position and repeat on the other side.

EXERCISE 2: GLUTES AND PIRIFORMIS STRETCH

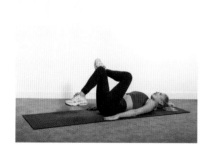
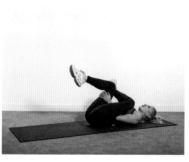

Still lying on your back, rest your left ankle on your right knee. Clasp your hands together behind your right leg, lift it slightly and pull towards you until you feel the stretch. Bring the left leg down and do the same to the other leg.

EXERCISE 3: SPINAL MOBILITY ROCK

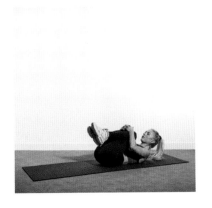
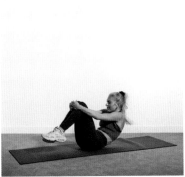

Lying on the floor, bring both knees in towards your chest. Rock forwards and backwards, with just small movements at first but incrementally increasing the range of motion, which is going to increase your flexibility through your spine.

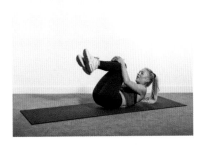
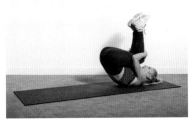

EXERCISE 4: LOWER LUMBAR WRING

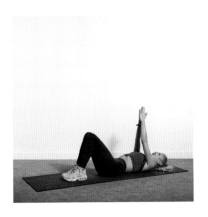
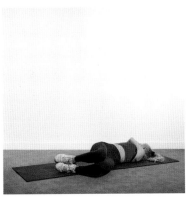

Still lying on your back, bend your knees and bring your heels close to your glutes. Extend your arms upwards and bring your palms together. Rock both legs in one direction while your arms move in the opposite direction in a wringing motion. Move from side to side metronomically.

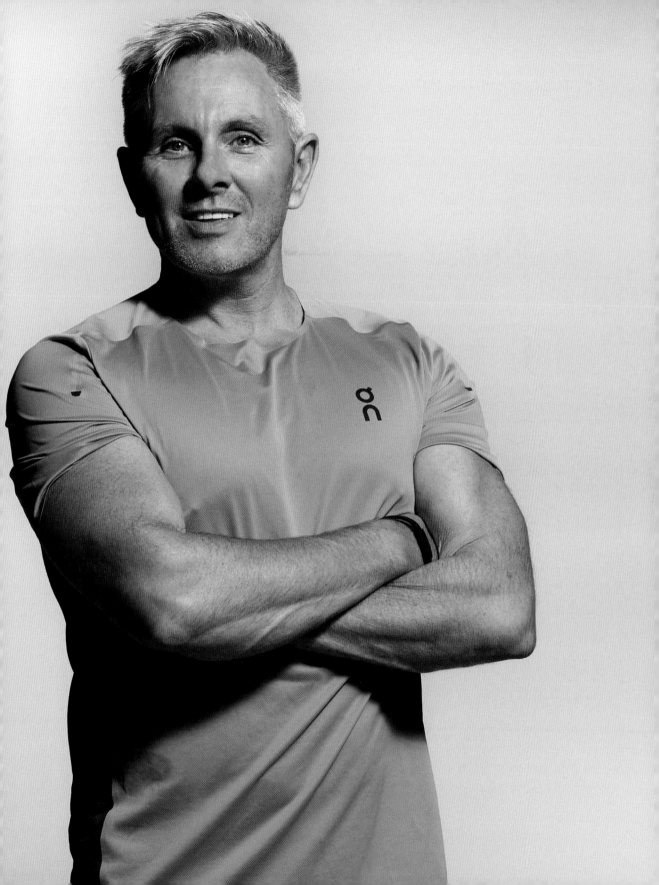

EXERCISE 5: UPPER-BODY MATRIX

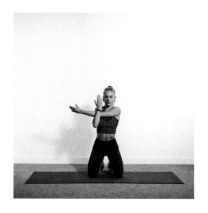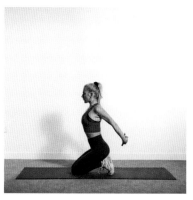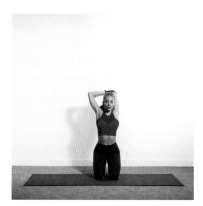

Kneel down and sit on your heels. Bring one arm across your body and hold it in place with the other. Pull your arm into your chest until you feel a comfortable stretch in your shoulder. Repeat the same movements with the other arm.

Now bring your arms behind your back and clasp your hands together. Raise your hands slightly, bringing them up and away from your body, pushing your chest out slightly.

Next, bring one arm up over your head and down the centre of your back, with your fingers pointing directly down your spine. Using your other hand, put a little bit of pressure on your elbow to stretch your triceps. Now do the same with the other arm.

BY NOW YOU SHOULD BE ENJOYING YOURSELF AND FEELING COMMITTED TO THE CHALLENGE.

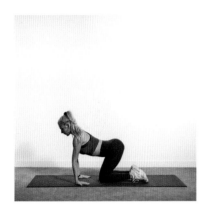
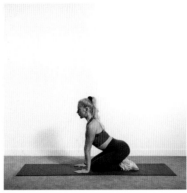

Still on your knees, place your palms on the floor, with your fingers pointing back towards you. You're stretching your forearms and leaning back slightly. Sit up and put your hands the other way around, with your fingers pointing in front of you. Then rotate the wrists clockwise and then anticlockwise.

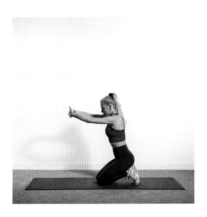

Clasping your hands together in front of you, push them away from you, with your shoulder blades open. Hold and then return to the start position.

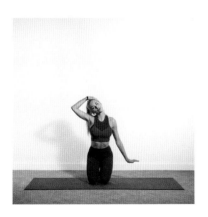

Put one hand over your head with your fingers touching the opposite side. You're applying enough pressure so your head drops to one side, giving yourself a comfortable neck stretch. Do the same with your other hand.

CORE

	10–15 REPS / 20–30 SECONDS
	15–20 REPS / 30–40 SECONDS
	20–25 REPS / 40–50 SECONDS

EXERCISE 1: WEIGHTED CRUNCHES

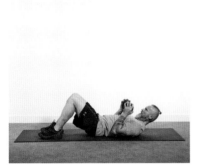 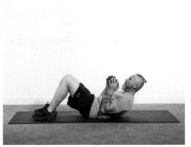 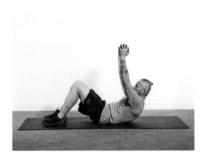

Lie on your back with your feet flat on the floor, holding a moderate dumbbell on your chest. Come up and squeeze your abdominals while maintaining a neutral back. Return to the start position.

If you're at a more advanced level, you have the option of raising the dumbbell above your head as you come up into the crunch.

EVERY EXERCISE SHOULD NOW START TO FEEL NATURAL RATHER THAN FORCED.

EXERCISE 2: WEIGHTED CRUNCHES WITH LEGS RAISED

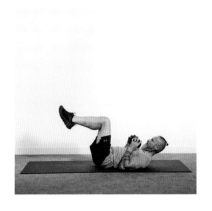 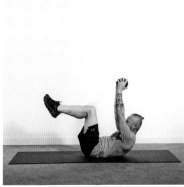

Still lying on your back, and still clasping a dumbbell on your chest, raise your legs into the air, bending your knees at 90 degrees. Lift your shoulders off the ground and lift the weight up above you with both hands. Return to the start position.

EXERCISE 3: V-SIT

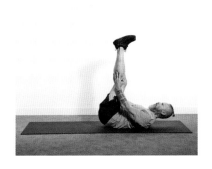 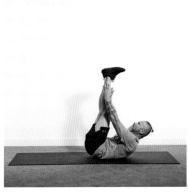

Lie on your back with your legs straight in the air at 90 degrees. Place your hands on the backs of both calves. Slide your hands up the back of your legs towards your feet as far as you comfortably can. Return to the start position.

EXERCISE 4: SIDE OBLIQUES

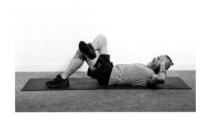 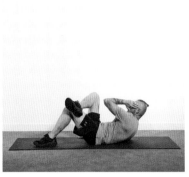

Cross your right leg over your left, with the ankle resting on the knee, and place your hands on your temples. Bring your left elbow over to meet your right knee, with your right arm on the ground. Now swap sides.

EXERCISE 5: ABDOMINAL WITH A HOLD

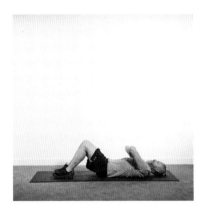 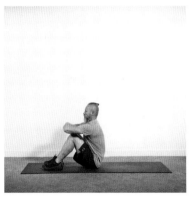 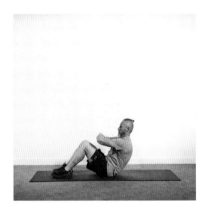

Lie on the floor with your forearms crossed above your chest and your knees bent. Raise yourself all the way up, until your arms meet your knees. Return to the mid-position, which is halfway between lying down and sitting up, and hold for five seconds with your arms still crossed. Return to the start position.

FULL BODY

	10–15 REPS / 20–30 SECONDS
	15–20 REPS / 30–40 SECONDS
	20–25 REPS / 40–50 SECONDS

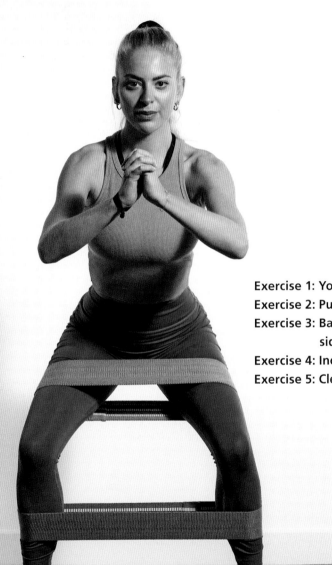

Exercise 1: Your weakest legs exercise

Exercise 2: Push-up with a knee drive (see page 97)

Exercise 3: Band matrix with a second band and extra side skips (see page 93)

Exercise 4: Incline single-arm dumbbells (see page 100)

Exercise 5: Clean and press (see page 41)

WEEK 4 RECAP

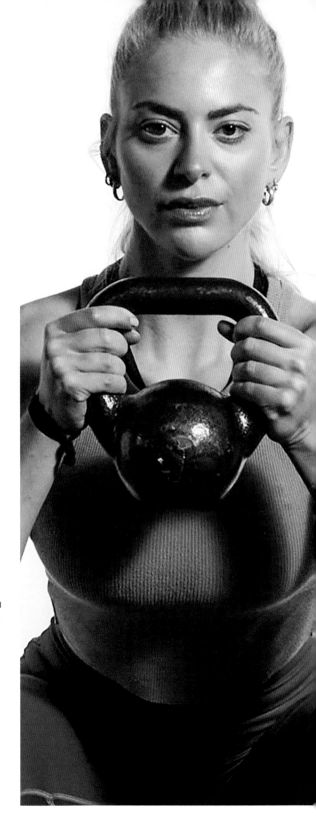

NUTRITION

○ People think that water is just for hydration, but it also gives you energy and clarity of thought before a workout. You don't always need a coffee or a snack for a pre-workout energy boost.

○ If you're training somewhere hot and humid and you're sweating a lot, you might want to add hydration tablets to your water, as they contain electrolytes and minerals.

○ If you're going to eat before a workout, around thirty minutes beforehand would be ideal as that gives the body time to prepare itself to do the task in hand. Don't eat a heavy meal; this should be an activation snack.

WELLBEING

○ If you're training at home or somewhere private, you could think about pinning something motivational to the wall, such as inspirational photos or a positive quote or message.

○ It helps to recognize that there's no quick fix with fitness, and that you have to put in the work if you want to achieve the goals you have set yourself.

○ Could you walk, run or cycle to your gym rather than driving or taking the bus or train? That would add to your fitness programme.

○ Don't be hard on yourself or push yourself to the extreme, as that won't be healthy for your body or brain.

ACCUMULATOR: 5–3

LEGS MONDAY	1: BOSU goblet squat 2: Band matrix with a second band and extra side skips 3: Sprinter lunge on the BOSU with resistance 4: Box jump with resistance 5: One-legged hip thrust with resistance
UPPER-BODY TUESDAY	1: Push-up with a knee drive 2: Shoulder matrix seated with half movements 3: Arms matrix seated 4: Incline single-arm dumbbells 5: Clean and press
DYNAMICS WEDNESDAY	1: Lower lumbar stretch 2: Glutes and piriformis stretch 3: Spinal mobility rock 4: Lower lumbar wring 5: Upper-body matrix
CORE THURSDAY	1: Weighted crunches 2: Weighted crunches with legs raised 3: V-Sit 4: Side obliques 5: Abdominal with a hold
FULL-BODY FRIDAY	1: Your weakest legs exercise 2: Push-up with a knee drive 3: Band matrix with a second band and extra side skips 4: Incline single-arm dumbbells 5: Clean and press
ACTIVE SATURDAY	Surprise and challenge your body by doing something for the first time. Is there a sport that have you always been interested in but you have never found the time to try it? Now's your moment.

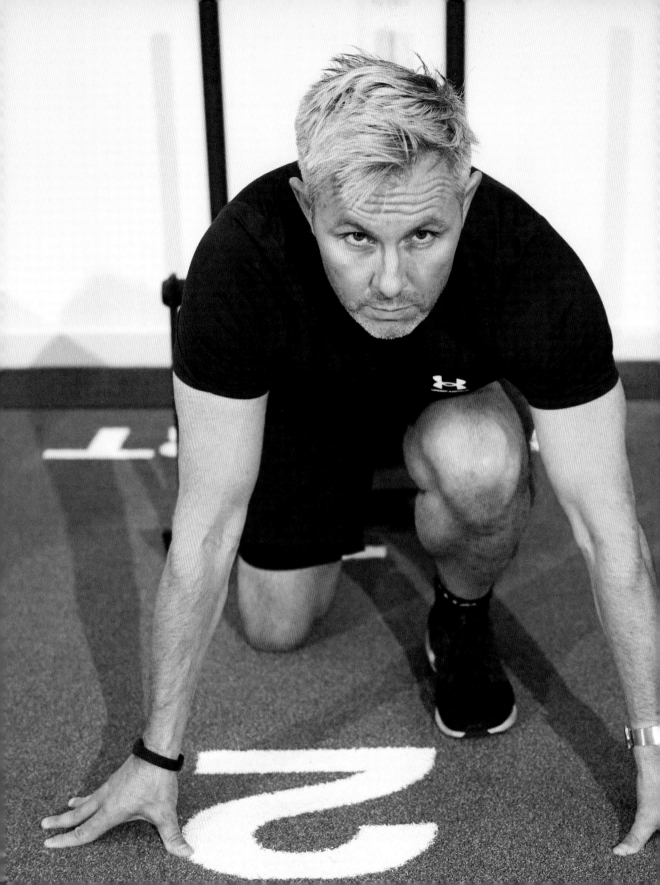

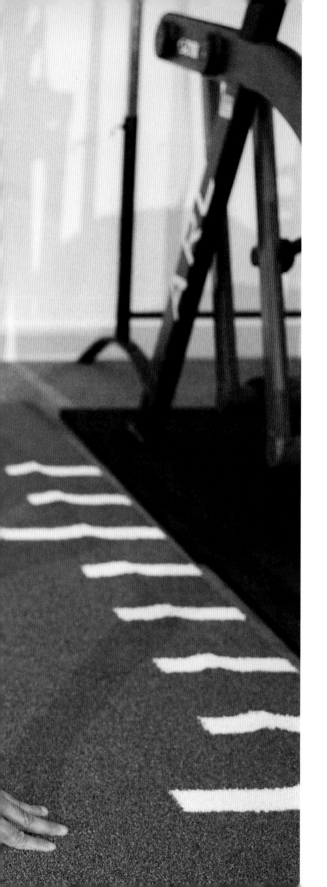

WEEK 5

'THIS DUDE IS LEGIT...
HE'S AWESOME.
READ ABOUT ALL HIS
SECRETS, ALL THE
DIFFERENT STARS
HE'S TURNED INTO
HEROES ... IT'LL
CHANGE YOUR LIFE.'
Chris Pratt

TRUST THE PROCESS

When you start to increase the intensity of your workouts, you're bound to be slightly more prone to injury. That's when you must listen even more attentively to your body. It's important to be able to identify the difference between muscle soreness from working out and pain from a potential injury.

ACCUMULATOR: 5–3

The last thing you want when you're training is an injury, which is why you should do all you can to prevent getting one (though, unfortunately, injuries do happen and you can't always avoid them). If you hurt yourself, you'll quickly lose most of the momentum you've built up so far, and it's more than likely you'll have to pause your challenge – I wouldn't recommend the macho approach of trying to push through the pain because that tends to make things worse. Staying healthy and consistent is the key to completing this ten-week challenge and getting the most from yourself.

By now, your recovery after exercise will be better than it was in Week 1. But your body will soon tell you if your programme is too intense. If you're increasing the intensity week on week, you could test out the exercises at the start of a new week for a day or two and see how you feel. If it doesn't feel quite right, or you're sorer than you had anticipated, you could consider going back to the exercises you were doing the week before. I've never bought into that mantra of 'no pain, no gain'. Being in pain should never be used as a metric. But feeling pain can often be useful. It alerts you to the fact that a certain part of your body is doing too much. Now you've got a chance to address that. Always listen to what your body is telling you and then react. If you're feeling tight in one area, or you've got a niggle, you need to address what that limb or muscle is saying rather than ignoring it and just pushing on.

BE FLEXIBLE

If you can be flexible about when you train different muscle groups, that will help you to avoid injury. So, for example, let's say your legs are still screaming from a workout you did a few days ago and you're supposed to be training them again today: you can always train your upper body instead. That ensures you maintain your momentum. If you're unsure whether a muscle is ready to train, test it by trying to contract it. If it won't contract, and it's not firing up at all (i.e. it's not waking up and activating), it possibly means it's fatigued and is still in a state of repair. You always have the option, if you're feeling extremely sore all over and it's all getting a bit too much, to give yourself some days off. And you should rest without feeling any guilt whatsoever, because taking a break will allow you to complete the ten weeks without creating any long-term health issues. But when you restart the challenge, ensure you go back and start the week from the beginning, so you're not missing a chunk of your programme.

WEEK 5 KIT LIST

BANDS
BAR AND WEIGHTS
BENCHES
BOSU
BOX
DUMBBELLS
SWISS BALL

HOW'S YOUR SLEEP?

I'm always asking actors I work with about their sleep. Your sleep will usually tell you if you're training and eating at the right level or if your intensity is too high and your nutrition is too low. If you're sleeping well, that's a strong indication that your body is coping. But if your sleep isn't great, that could be because you're asking too much of your body with the workouts, or you're being hard on yourself with the nutrition, or possibly even both. Broken sleep can affect your energy and concentration, and as a result you might not pay so much attention to your form, increasing the risk of getting injured. And don't forget to stretch. Stretching will reduce the chance of injury.

LISTEN, FEEL, UNDERSTAND, REACT. ALWAYS LISTEN TO YOUR BODY AND REACT TO WHAT IT'S TELLING YOU.

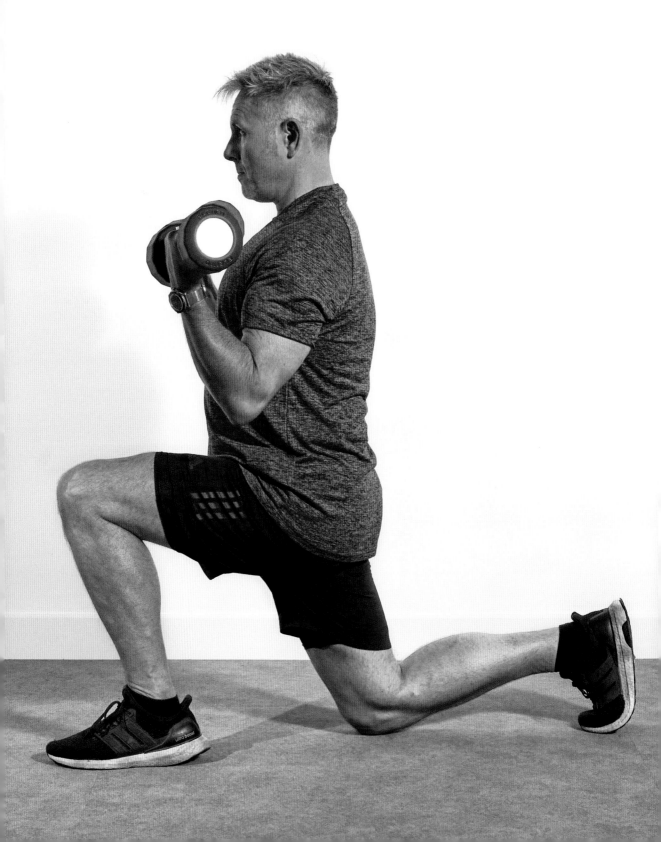

LEGS

EXERCISE 1: SQUAT WITH A JUMP

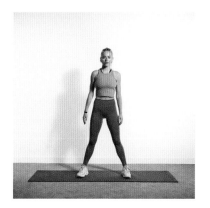 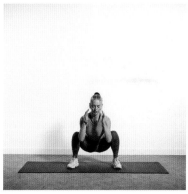 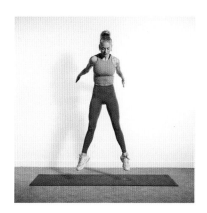

Stand with your feet shoulder-width apart, and your toes pointing slightly outwards. Lower yourself down until your knees are at 90 degrees and hold that position for a count of four. Explode through your heels to standing. Jump into the air and return to the start postion.

EXERCISE 2: BAND MATRIX WITH A SECOND BAND AND EXTRA SIDE SKIPS (SEE PAGE 93)

EXERCISE 3: BALLISTIC LUNGE

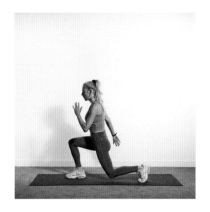 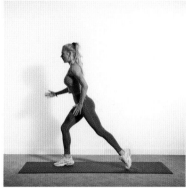 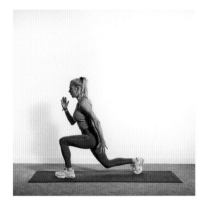

Stand with your feet shoulder-width apart. Lunge forward, dropping your rear leg until your knee kisses the floor. Push up, returning to the start position. Do a skip and switch to the other leg, and now do the same on the other side.

REMEMBER TO STRETCH – THERE'S NEVER ANY HARM IN DOING ADDITIONAL STRETCHING ROUTINES AROUND YOUR WORKOUT.

EXERCISE 4: BOX JUMP WITH A SQUAT

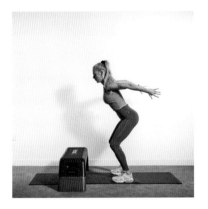 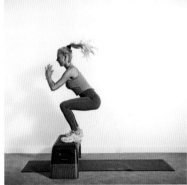 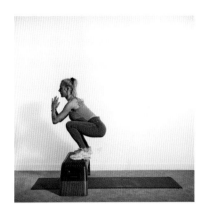

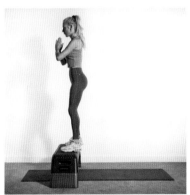 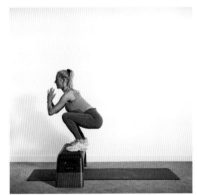 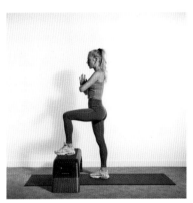

Stand 10 inches or 25 centimetres back from the box with your feet shoulder-width apart and your arms by your sides. Get into a squat position and then propel yourself through the air, landing with both feet on the box. Do a squat on top of the box. Step down from the box and return to the start position.

EXERCISE 5: HIP THRUST WITH A BAND

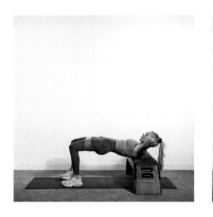 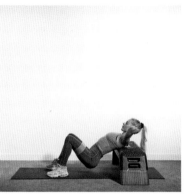

With a band around your knees, lie back with your shoulder blades on a bench, your knees at 90 degrees and your feet shoulder-width apart. Lower your glutes until they're about an inch or 2.5 centimetres off the ground. With control, return to the start position while contracting the glutes.

I KNOW PEOPLE DON'T ALWAYS LOVE LEGS DAY. THAT'S WHY DOING IT ON A MONDAY HELPS. YOU'VE GOT IT OVER AND DONE WITH!

UPPER BODY

10–15 REPS / 20–30 SECONDS
15–20 REPS / 30–40 SECONDS
20–25 REPS / 40–50 SECONDS

EXERCISE 1: PUSH-UP WITH A CLAP

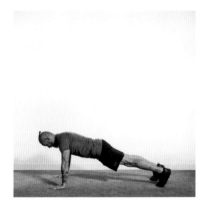
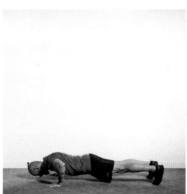

Place your hands on the ground, shoulder-width apart. Lower yourself down until your elbows are at 90 degrees. Push up, breathing out on exertion, using enough power to lift your hands off the ground. Clap your hands together in the air. Return to the start position.

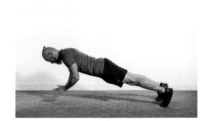
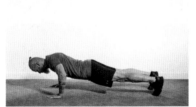

EXERCISE 2: SHOULDER MATRIX ON A SWISS BALL

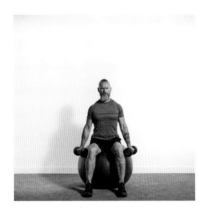 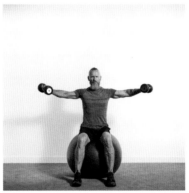

Seated on a Swiss ball, you can't use your legs and you're isolating the upper body. For the lateral raises, lift the dumbbells to the side with slightly bent elbows so they are level with your shoulders. Return to the start position.

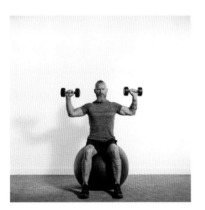 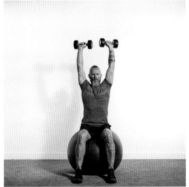

Transition from lateral raises into a shoulder press. Hold the dumbbells so that your arms are at 90 degrees on either side and the dumbbells are about 6 inches or 15 centimetres away from your ears. Raise the dumbbells into the air and then bring them together so they gently kiss. Bring them back down so your elbows and arms are at 90 degrees once again.

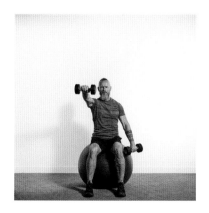 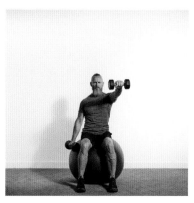

Transition into forward raises. Hold the dumbbells so they are touching your thighs and then lift one dumbbell up with a slightly bent elbow to shoulder height and return to the start position. Repeat on the other side.

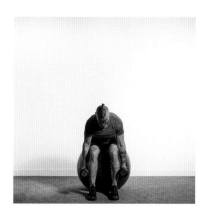 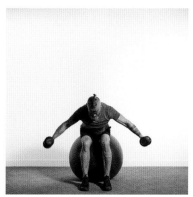

Transition into a bent-over row. Maintain a neutral spine, back and neck. The dumbbells are dangling in front of you beneath your chest and by your shins. With a slight bend in your elbows, retract the dumbbells so they are parallel with your shoulders and then return to the start position.

EXERCISE 3: ARMS MATRIX ON A SWISS BALL

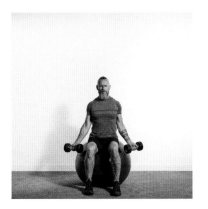 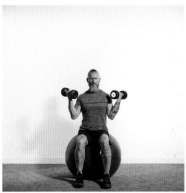

You're sitting down on a Swiss ball, which isolates the muscles. Hold a dumbbell in each hand so they are about 6 inches or 15 centimetres away from your legs, with your palms facing away from your body. Slowly raise your dumbbells up to shoulder height. Lift your elbows a couple of inches or 5 centimetres higher for extra pressure and then return to the start position.

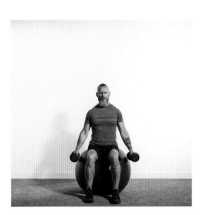 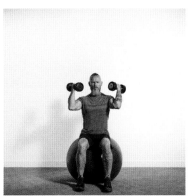

Change the hand position so your palms are now facing your body and the dumbbells are close to your legs. Curl the dumbbells up to shoulder height and then, with a little tip of the elbows which applies extra pressure on the bicep, return to the start position.

You'll need a bench for triceps dips (see pages 39 and 66 for photos). For added resistance, use two benches and raise your legs. You should almost be sitting on your hands, with your fingers coming off the edge of the bench. Lower yourself down until your elbows are at 90 degrees. Return to the start position.

EXERCISE 4: BOSU BENT-OVER ROW WITH DOUBLE DUMBBELLS

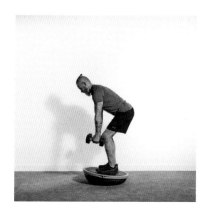 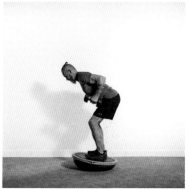

Standing on the BOSU, hard side up, bend over slightly with a neutral back while holding a moderate dumbbell in each hand. Lift the weights at the same time towards your chest and then lower them to the start position.

EXERCISE 5: CLEAN AND PRESS (SEE PAGE 41)

DON'T FEEL INTIMIDATED OR EMBARRASSED ABOUT USING UNFAMILIAR BITS OF KIT. VARIETY IS SO IMPORTANT.

DYNAMIC STRETCHING

	10–15 REPS / 20–30 SECONDS
	15–20 REPS / 30–40 SECONDS
	20–25 REPS / 40–50 SECONDS

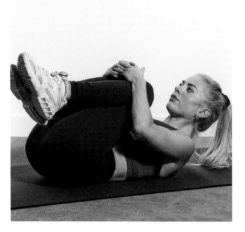

Exercise 1: Lower lumbar stretch (see page 101)
Exercise 2: Glutes and piriformis stretch (see page 101)
Exercise 3: Spinal mobility rock (see page 102)
Exercise 4: Lower lumbar wring (see page 102)
Exercise 5: Upper-body matrix (see page 104)

WEEK 5 / **THURSDAY**

CORE

	10–15 REPS / 20–30 SECONDS
	15–20 REPS / 30–40 SECONDS
	20–25 REPS / 40–50 SECONDS

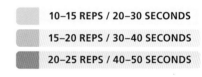

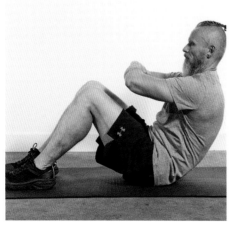

Exercise 1: Weighted crunches (see page 106)
Exercise 2: Weighted crunches with legs
 raised (see page 107)
Exercise 3: V-Sit (see page 107)
Exercise 4: Side obliques (see page 108)
Exercise 5: Abdominal with a hold (see page 108)

FULL BODY

10–15 REPS / 20–30 SECONDS
15–20 REPS / 30–40 SECONDS
20–25 REPS / 40–50 SECONDS

Exercise 1: Your weakest legs exercise
Exercise 2: Push-up with a clap (see page 121)
Exercise 3: Band matrix with a second band and extra side skips (see page 93)
Exercise 4: BOSU bent-over row with double dumbbells (see page 125)
Exercise 5: Clean and press (see page 41)

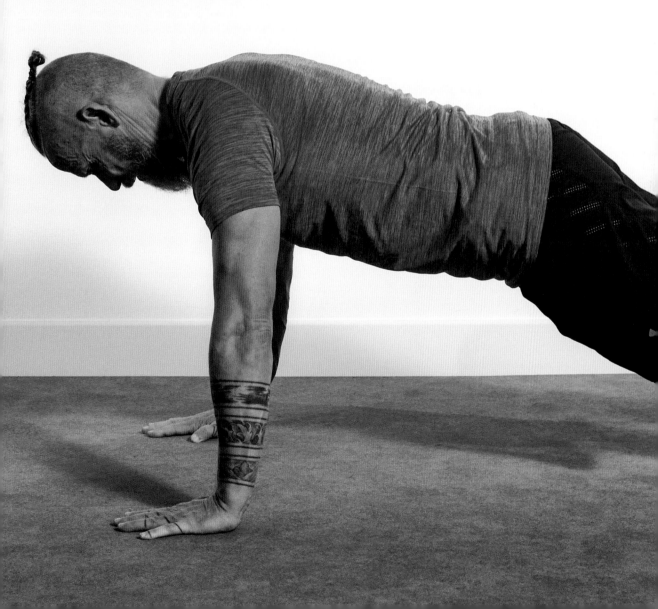

WEEK 5 RECAP

NUTRITION

O Sipping water between exercises is OK, but don't take an extended water break because then you will lose some of your intensity and your heart rate will start to come down.

O The colour of your urine during the day is a good indication of whether you're hydrated enough. It should almost be clear.

O Some people like to drink water during the night. The body will get into a pattern of wanting a drink at around the same time every night. While that can help with your hydration, the downside is that it's disrupting your sleep.

O Before you eat anything, ask yourself: 'What will this food do for me and why am I having it now?' Always look for options that are nutritous as well as energy-boosting.

WELLBEING

O Always take any opportunity to get into water, whether it's a pool or the sea, as it's great for de-stressing your body and amazing for your wellbeing.

O Think carefully before deciding whether to step on the scales because if you don't like the number you see, will that ruin your mood for the rest of the day? You're working hard and your body is changing, but that won't necessarily be reflected in your weight.

O Focus on body composition rather than weight. Remember that muscle weighs more than fat.

O Talk to yourself in a positive way. Tell yourself before a workout, 'I will do this,' and afterwards say, 'I have done this,' as that will help to give you a sense of achievement.

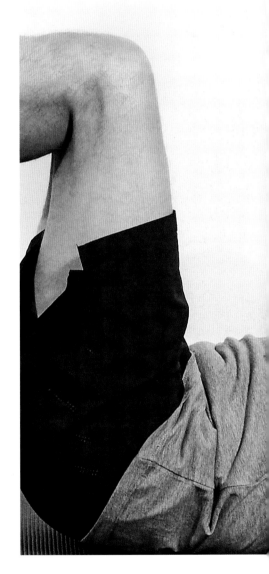

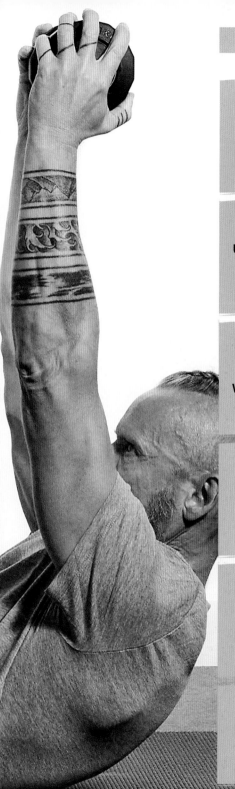

LEGS MONDAY	1: Squat with a jump 2: Band matrix with a second band and extra side skips 3: Ballistic lunge 4: Box jump with a squat 5: Hip thrust with a band
UPPER-BODY TUESDAY	1: Push-up with a clap 2: Shoulder matrix on a Swiss ball 3: Arms matrix on a Swiss ball 4: BOSU bent-over row with double dumbbells 5: Clean and press
DYNAMICS WEDNESDAY	1: Lower lumbar stretch 2: Glutes and piriformis stretch 3: Spinal mobility rock 4: Lower lumbar wring 5: Upper-body matrix
CORE THURSDAY	1: Weighted crunches 2: Weighted crunches with legs raised 3: V-Sit 4: Side obliques 5: Abdominal with a hold
FULL-BODY FRIDAY	1: Your weakest legs exercise 2: Push-up with a clap 3: Band matrix with a second band and extra side skips 4: BOSU bent-over row with double dumbbells 5: Clean and press
ACTIVE SATURDAY	Is there a sport you enjoy watching? Take some inspiration from those athletes involved. For instance, that could mean getting out on the tennis or basketball court.

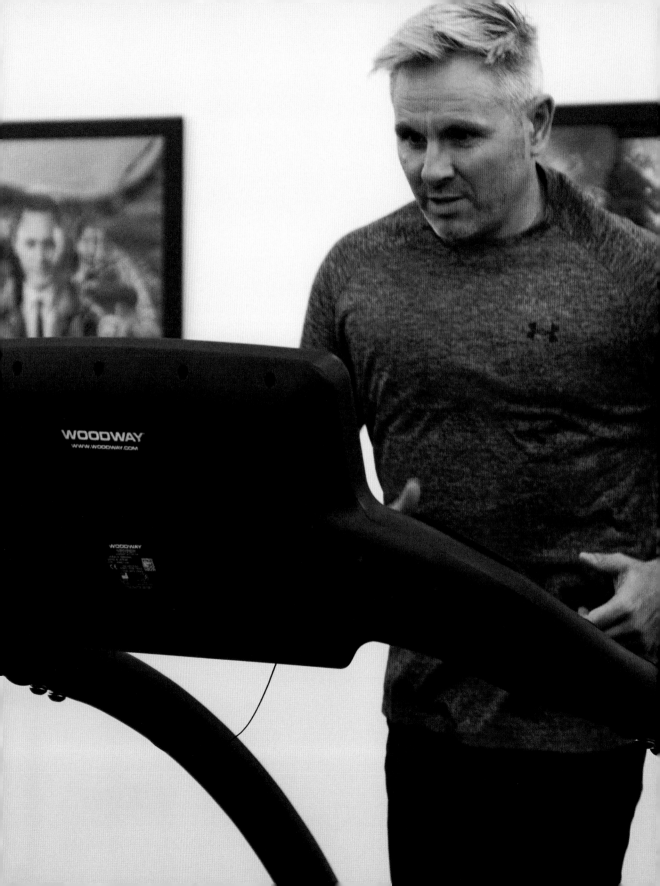

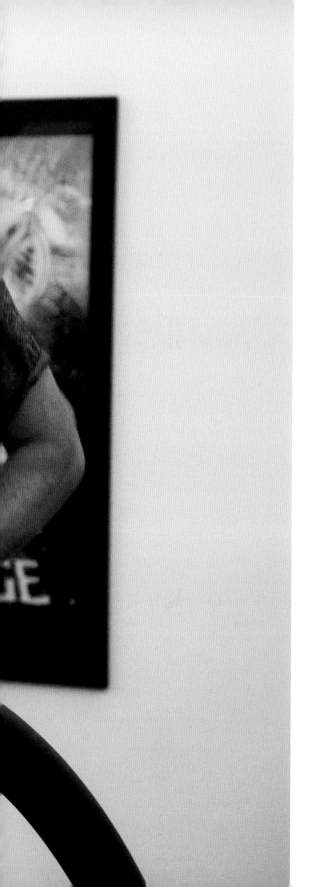

WEEK 6

'I OWE SO MUCH
TO SIMON. HIS
FRIENDSHIP AND
GUIDANCE SAW
ME THROUGH
MANY PHYSICAL
CHALLENGES.'
Daniel Craig

IT'S MAKE OR BREAK

If you're thinking that you want to quit at this point in the challenge, you're certainly not alone. This is notoriously the moment, six weeks in, when lots of people are checking out. Don't be a quitter!

ACCUMULATOR: 5–3

I believe that around 90 per cent of people who have embarked on a new fitness programme consider abandoning it at the six-week mark. If you're doubting yourself, and struggling for motivation, it might help you to know that it's perfectly normal to have such a mindset, and you're certainly not alone in feeling that way at this moment.

You might be thinking that you're not making as much progress as you would like to, that you're plateauing. It's possibly the hardest part of the programme, so be prepared to feel this way and talk yourself around. After all your efforts to get to

this point, don't let yourself be another person who started with so much motivation only for it to fizzle out before completing the ten weeks. You might want to use the knowledge that this is a common time to drop the programme as a motivator – be energized by the desire not to be another Week-6 quitter.

KEEP GOING
Consider how much you have already accomplished. You've got this deep into the programme so don't throw all of that away. Perhaps you're wondering whether you've already done enough and seen some benefits, and you're starting to prioritize other

parts of your life. While it's true you'll now be fitter than you were at the start of this challenge, and you should be feeling better, aren't you curious about how much more you could achieve? I can assure you that if you get through this week, and move on to Week 7 and beyond, you're about to see some serious results. Your progress is about to speed up. If you step away now, you'll miss out on all of that. While some people want to stop this week, others find that this is when they get super motivated. Which way will you go?

BE POSITIVE

To help you get you through this week, feel free to talk to yourself in a super-positive and motivational way. I use very upbeat and encouraging language when speaking to a client who is in Week 6. I'll be saying: 'Day forty, this is the best day ever! One day at a time. We're on it.' I'm always telling my clients that they're having an amazing week. Can you be just as optimistic and constructive with yourself? Talking to like-minded people and explaining how you feel will also help, as they might have some supportive words to keep you going.

WEEK 6 KIT LIST

BANDS
BOSU
BOX
DUMBBELLS
SWISS BALL

You also might want to consider dropping the intensity by 10 per cent, through doing slightly fewer reps or selecting lighter weights, or even a combination of the two. If your workouts are a little easier, you're more likely to feel good about yourself and how your challenge is going. If you recognize that you're on the right track, you won't want to quit. For extra stimulation, you could even try doing different cardio. Keeping it fresh always helps.

THIS IS *MEANT* TO BE CHALLENGING – THERE ARE GOING TO BE TOUGH MOMENTS ALONG THE WAY, BUT YOU CAN GET THROUGH THEM.

LEGS

10–15 REPS / 20–30 SECONDS	
15–20 REPS / 30–40 SECONDS	
20–25 REPS / 40–50 SECONDS	

EXERCISE 1: SQUAT WITH A BAND

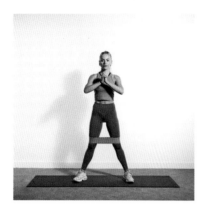
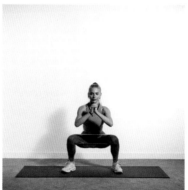

Place a resistance band just above your knees. Your feet are shoulder-width apart, with your toes pointing slightly outwards. Lower yourself down until your knees are at 90 degrees and hold that position for a count of four. Push up through your heels to return to the start position.

EXERCISE 2: BAND MATRIX WITH A SECOND BAND AND EXTRA SIDE SKIPS (SEE PAGE 93)

EXERCISE 3: REVERSE LUNGE

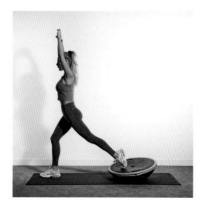
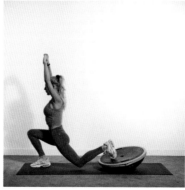

Stand with your feet shoulder-width apart and your arms above your head, hands locked and palms facing forwards. Lunge backwards, placing one foot on the hard side of a BOSU and dropping your knee towards the floor. Explode upwards, returning to the start position. Do the reps on the same side and then switch legs.

EXERCISE 4: BOX JUMP WITH A SQUAT AND RESISTANCE

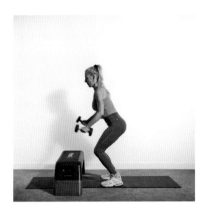 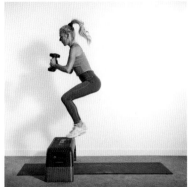

Holding dumbbells, stand 10 inches or 25 centimetres back from the box with your feet shoulder-width apart and your arms by your sides. Get into a squat position. Propel yourself through the air and bring the dumbbells together as you land with both feet on the box. Do a squat on top of the box, then step down.

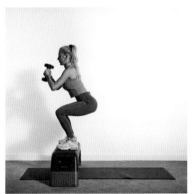 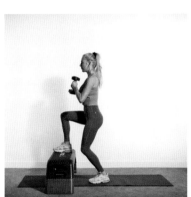

ENSURE YOUR INNER VOICE IS ALWAYS POSITIVE AND ENCOURAGING.

EXERCISE 5: HIP THRUST WITH A BAND AND RESISTANCE

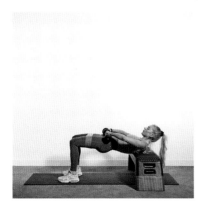 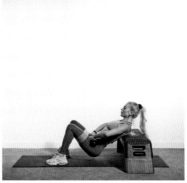

With a band around your knees and two dumbbells resting across your hips, lie back with your shoulder blades on the bench, your knees at 90 degrees and your feet shoulder-width apart. Lower your glutes until they're about an inch or 2.5 centimetres off the ground. With control, return to the start position while contracting the glutes.

VISUALIZATION HELPS. PICTURE IN YOUR MIND WHAT YOU'RE ABOUT TO DO AND WHERE YOU'RE GOING – SEE YOURSELF GETTING THERE.

UPPER BODY

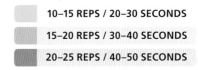

10–15 REPS / 20–30 SECONDS

15–20 REPS / 30–40 SECONDS

20–25 REPS / 40–50 SECONDS

EXERCISE 1: SWITCH HAND PUSH-UP

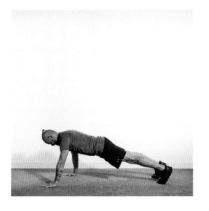

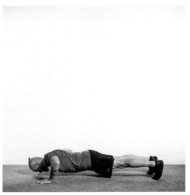

Place your hands on the ground, shoulder-width apart, with one hand slightly in front of the other. Lower yourself down until your elbows are at 90 degrees. Push up, breathing out on exertion, and switch your hands so the other one is slightly in front before the next rep.

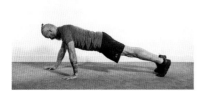

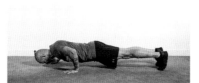

EXERCISE 2: SHOULDER MATRIX ON A SWISS BALL WITH HALF MOVEMENTS

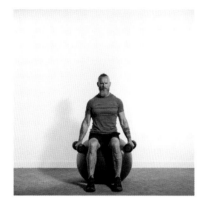 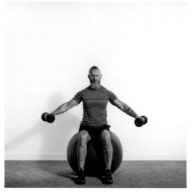

Seated on a Swiss ball, you can't use your legs and you're isolating the upper body. You're doing half movements for the lateral raises, which means the muscles are under constant tension. For the lateral raises, lift the dumbbells to the side with slightly bent elbows, so they are halfway to being level with your shoulders. Return to the start position.

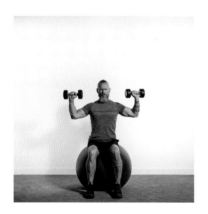 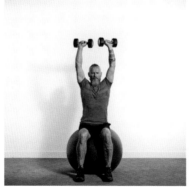

Transition from lateral raises into a shoulder press. Hold the dumbbells so that your arms are at 90 degrees on either side and the dumbbells are about 6 inches or 15 centimetres away from your ears. Raise the dumbbells into the air and then bring them together so they gently kiss. Bring them back down so your elbows and arms are at 90 degrees once again.

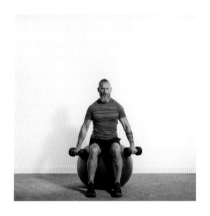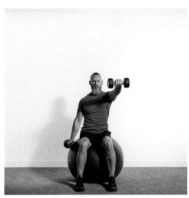

Transition into forward double raises. Hold the dumbbells so they are touching your thighs and then lift one dumbbell up with a slightly bent elbow to shoulder height, and return to the start position. Repeat on the other side.

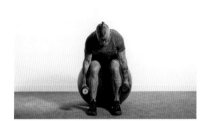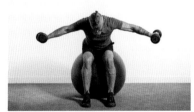

Transition into a bent-over row. Maintain a neutral spine, back and neck. The dumbbells are dangling in front of you beneath your chest and by your shins. With a slight bend in your elbows, retract the dumbbells so they are level with your shoulders and then return to the start position.

EXERCISE 3: ARMS MATRIX ON A SWISS BALL (SEE PAGE 124)

EXERCISE 4: BOSU ALTERNATE BENT-OVER ROW WITH DUMBBELLS

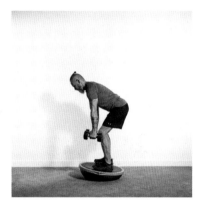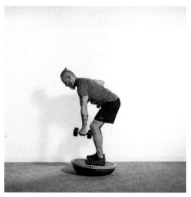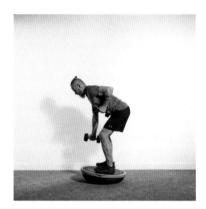

Standing on the BOSU, bend over slightly while holding a moderate dumbbell in each hand. Lift one weight at a time towards your chest and then lower to the start position. Now do the same on the other side.

EXERCISE 5: CLEAN AND PRESS WITH DUMBBELLS

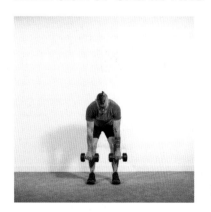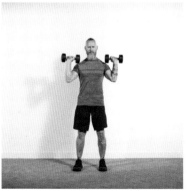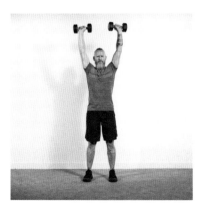

Holding two dumbbells, bend down into the squat position with your knees slightly soft. The weights should be halfway between your knees and ankles. Drive up the squat, raise dumbbells to your shoulders and then press the dumbbells into the air.

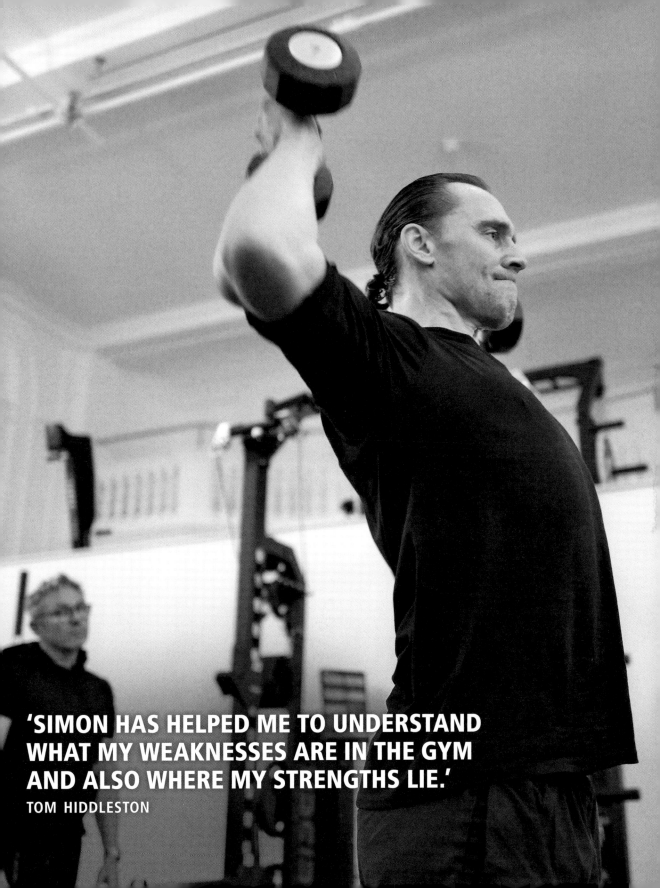

'SIMON HAS HELPED ME TO UNDERSTAND
WHAT MY WEAKNESSES ARE IN THE GYM
AND ALSO WHERE MY STRENGTHS LIE.'
TOM HIDDLESTON

DYNAMIC STRETCHING

	10–15 REPS / 20–30 SECONDS
	15–20 REPS / 30–40 SECONDS
	20–25 REPS / 40–50 SECONDS

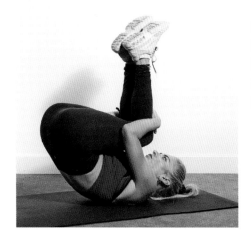

Exercise 1: Lower lumbar stretch (see page 101)
Exercise 2: Glutes and piriformis stretch (see page 101)
Exercise 3: Spinal mobility rock (see page 102)
Exercise 4: Lower lumbar wring (see page 102)
Exercise 5: Upper-body matrix (see page 104)

WEEK 6 / **THURSDAY**

CORE

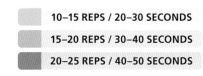

	10–15 REPS / 20–30 SECONDS
	15–20 REPS / 30–40 SECONDS
	20–25 REPS / 40–50 SECONDS

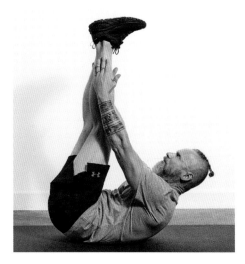

Exercise 1: Weighted crunches (see page 106)
Exercise 2: Weighted crunches with legs raised
            (see page 107)
Exercise 3: V-Sit (see page 107)
Exercise 4: Side obliques (see page 108)
Exercise 5: Abdominal with a hold (see page 108)

FULL BODY

Exercise 1: Your weakest legs exercise

Exercise 2: Switch hand push-up (see page 137)

Exercise 3: Band matrix with a second band and extra side skips (see page 93)

Exercise 4: BOSU alternate bent-over row with dumbbells (see page 140)

Exercise 5: Clean and press with dumbbells (see page 140)

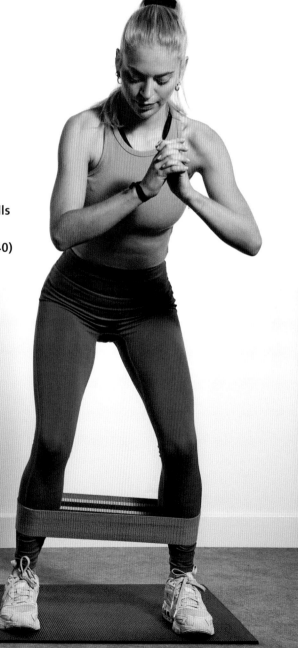

WEEK 6 RECAP

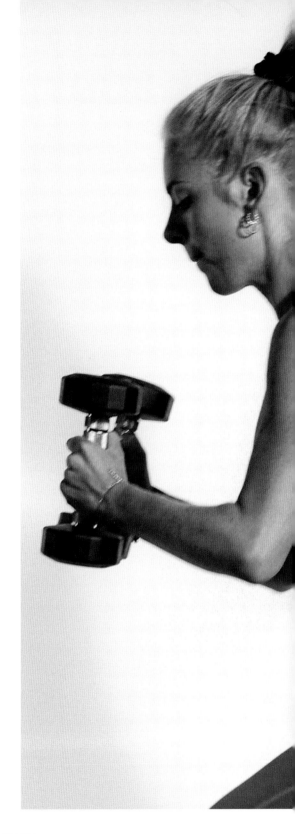

NUTRITION

○ If you're really craving something, go ahead and have it, albeit in moderation. Don't be too restrictive or hard on yourself.

○ Being prepared is key to avoiding temptation. When you're very hungry, you're going to pick up the first thing you can. But if you've planned ahead sufficiently well and you have fresh, healthy ingredients in your fridge, you can make yourself something more nutritious.

○ If you're putting in the effort to make something healthy to eat, why not double up with the ingredients in order to have the same meal ready to enjoy again tomorrow or later in the week?

WELLBEING

○ If you're feeling low on energy and motivation at any point this week, and you don't feel as though you can possibly do the whole workout, just get started. Once you've done that, and your body and mind get going, you might surprise yourself.

○ After you have worked out, do you feel as though you want to snooze on the sofa or are you feeling full of energy? Exercise should re-energize you and set you up for the day.

○ Having a more positive outlook on life will help you to feel good and it will also allow you to progress your fitness, as you'll understand that you're on the right path towards some encouraging results.

ACCUMULATOR: 5–3

LEGS MONDAY	1: Squat with a band 2: Band matrix with a second band and extra side skips 3: Reverse lunge 4: Box jump with a squat and resistance 5: Hip thrust with a band and resistance
UPPER-BODY TUESDAY	1: Switch hand push-up 2: Shoulder matrix on a Swiss ball with half movements 3: Arms matrix on a Swiss ball 4: BOSU alternate bent-over row with dumbbells 5: Clean and press with dumbbells
DYNAMICS WEDNESDAY	1: Lower lumbar stretch 2: Glutes and piriformis stretch 3: Spinal mobility rock 4: Lower lumbar wring 5: Upper-body matrix
CORE THURSDAY	1: Weighted crunches 2: Weighted crunches with legs raised 3: V-Sit 4: Side obliques 5: Abdominal with a hold
FULL-BODY FRIDAY	1: Your weakest legs exercise 2: Switch hand push-up 3: Band matrix with a second band and extra side skips 4: BOSU alternate bent-over row with dumbbells 5: Clean and press with dumbbells
ACTIVE SATURDAY	Do something that makes you feel alive. When was the last time you sprinted – and I mean really sprinted – rather than going for a fast jog? You could also ride your bike or kick a football around.

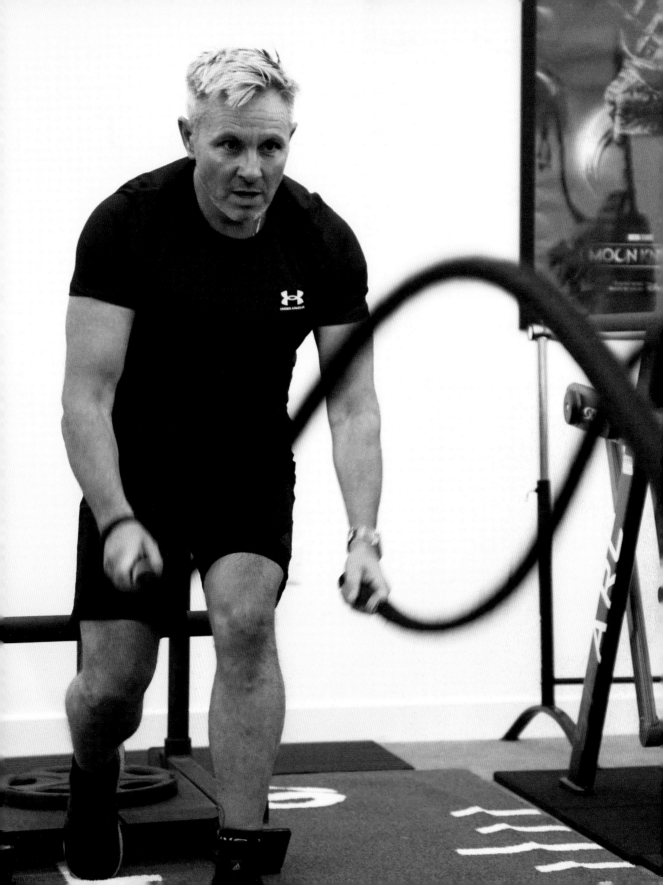

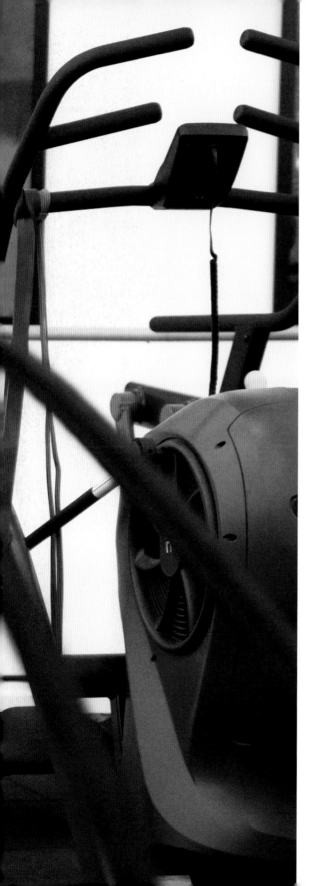

WEEK 7

'WITH SIMON'S HELP, I'VE BEEN ABLE TO SUSTAIN THE HIGHEST LEVELS OF HEALTH AND FITNESS THROUGH SEVERAL MOVIE FRANCHISES WITHOUT INJURY.'

Bryce Dallas Howard

ON TRACK

You mustn't ever feel guilty about missing a workout. So long as you have a good reason not to do the session that day – perhaps you've suddenly got a busy day at work or you have an important family occasion to attend – never feel guilty. Just ensure you'll be back at it tomorrow.

ACCUMULATOR: 5–4

Missing a workout because something unavoidable has come up is quite different to skipping a workout because you can't be bothered, or because you're a little tired or low on motivation and you would rather spend an hour doing something else. That's not OK. But if you can justify your decision not to train, you shouldn't feel bad that you have a life outside your programme. You have to be realistic and you have to be flexible.

Once you have got to this stage of the challenge, you have already set your trajectory, both mentally and physically, so if you miss a day here or there for good reason, don't feel as though you have lost everything you have been working so hard

for. You've already completed six weeks, so there's nothing to feel guilty about. You're already winning. You're not going to spiral out of the programme just because you missed one workout, so you shouldn't beat yourself up about it, as that's not going to make you feel good. Remember that this challenge is about enhancing your mental wellbeing as well as your physicality.

SHIFTING PRIORITIES
We all wish we could give 100 per cent to everything we do, including a fitness challenge, but life's not always like that. Everyone's priorities are constantly shifting, often from one day to the next, so it's OK when your work or family life are

taking more of your time, but always remember your fitness goal, and how you have challenged yourself to complete these ten weeks. Back in Week 2, I wrote about how athletes know how to self-manage, pulling back when needed and pushing when they can, and that's something to consider in this situation. Perhaps you've got a couple of days off coming up when you'll have the chance to push again, and maybe you've got a clear weekend and you can invest a little more time in your active recovery and wellness. But don't get carried away and try to significantly increase the intensity in your next few sessions, because by doing too much you'll risk injury. And if you hurt yourself, you'll miss more than one session: you'll have to put your challenge on pause.

In this week's workouts, I'm increasing your cardio between exercises from three minutes to four. Your cardiovascular system is becoming more efficient with every week and you should now be capable of doing another minute. Weeks 7, 8 and 9 are an opportunity to turn on the afterburners and to accelerate your progression. I'm introducing new dynamic stretching and core exercises this week. To help keep you stimulated and engaged, I'm also giving you some choice with your core workout on Thursday.

COUNTDOWN

If you're an actor and I'm preparing you for a part, you'll be on countdown now. You were given ten weeks to get ready for a particular role or sequence. The first six weeks, we would normally be left alone. But now the production team will be interested in your capability, such as your strength and agility. When we're about three or four weeks away from shooting, actors are normally also doing stunt

WEEK 7 KIT LIST

BAND
BENCHES
BOSU
BOX
DUMBBELLS
MEDICINE BALL (or other resistance item)

OPTIONAL
(for core variety)
CAGE
KETTLEBELL
SWISS BALL

choreography rehearsals, hair and make-up tests, and their costumes are being adjusted. In the same way, you should be considering what you want to accomplish in the final weeks. Take some time to consider what you're trying to get out of them.

LEGS

10–15 REPS / 20–30 SECONDS
15–20 REPS / 30–40 SECONDS
20–25 REPS / 40–50 SECONDS

EXERCISE 1: SQUAT WITH A BAND AND RESISTANCE

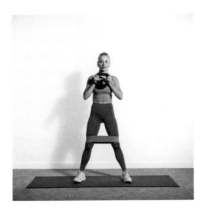 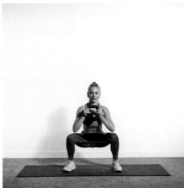

Put a resistance band just above your knees. Hold a kettlebell or other resistance item to your chest. Your feet are shoulder-width apart, with your toes pointing slightly outwards. Lower yourself down until your knees are at 90 degrees and hold that position for a count of four. Push up through your heels to return to the start position.

EXERCISE 2: WEIGHTED SIDE LUNGE WITH A KNEE DRIVE

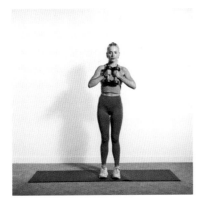 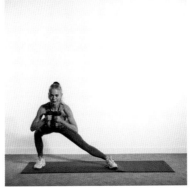 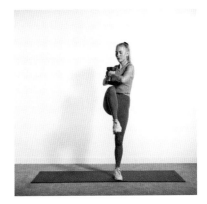

Hold dumbbells or a kettlebell to the middle of your chest. Take a step to your right and then go into a squat position on that side while keeping your left leg straight. Pushing through the heel, return to the start position and transition straight into a knee drive, raising your knee 90 degrees out in front of you, and twist your upper body round to the right. Return to the start position and repeat on the other leg.

EXERCISE 3: REVERSE LUNGE WITH RESISTANCE

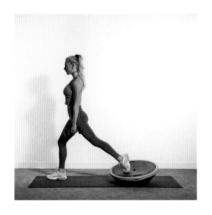
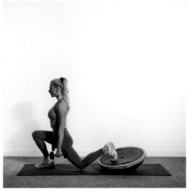

Stand with your feet shoulder-width apart, holding dumbbells or a kettlebell. Lunge backwards, placing your foot on the hard side of a BOSU and dropping your knee towards the floor. Explode upwards, returning to the start position. Do the reps on one leg and then switch legs.

EXERCISE 4: PLYOMETRIC BOX JUMP

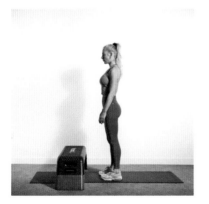
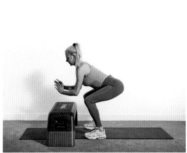

Stand 10 inches or 25 centimetres back from the box with your feet shoulder-width apart and your arms by your sides. Get into a squat position. Propel yourself through the air and land with both feet on the box. Then step down from the box. Now put your hands on the box, shoot your legs back and then forwards, and return to the start position.

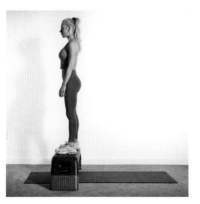
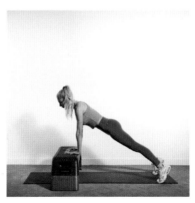

EXERCISE 5: ADAPTED NORDICS

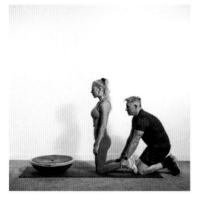
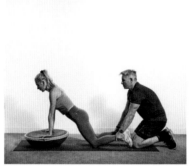

You're in a kneeling position but with your heels tucked under something, like a bench. If you have a training partner, ask them to hold your legs. With a BOSU or step in front of you, lower yourself down gradually, keeping your glutes and hamstrings tight, until your hands hit the BOSU or step – then lower yourself down until your elbows are at 90 degrees. Push yourself up, returning to the start position.

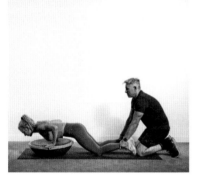
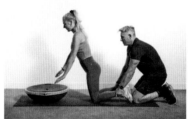

UPPER BODY

10–15 REPS / 20–30 SECONDS
15–20 REPS / 30–40 SECONDS
20–25 REPS / 40–50 SECONDS

EXERCISE 1: SWITCH HAND PUSH-UP WITH A KNEE DRIVE

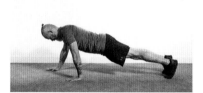 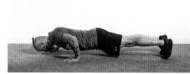 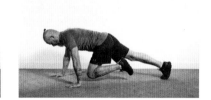

Place your hands on the ground shoulder-width apart, with one hand slightly in front of the other. Lower yourself down until your elbows are at 90 degrees. Push up, breathing out on exertion, and switch your hands so the other one is slightly in front. Drive your knee forward, alternating between the legs.

ACCEPT THAT YOUR PRIORITIES ARE CONSTANTLY SHIFTING AND THAT YOU'LL HAVE TO MISS A WORKOUT WHEN SOMETHING REALLY IMPORTANT COMES UP.

EXERCISE 2: SHOULDER MATRIX ON YOUR KNEES

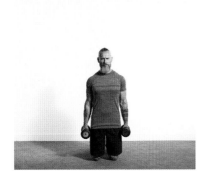 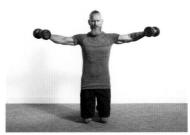

In a kneeling position, you can't use your legs and you're isolating the upper body. For the lateral raises, lift the dumbbells to the side with slightly bent elbows so they are level with your shoulders, and then return to the start position.

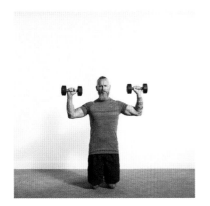 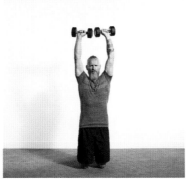

Transition from lateral raises into a shoulder press. Hold the dumbbells so that your arms are at 90 degrees on either side and the dumbbells are about 6 inches or 15 centimetres away from your ears. Raise the dumbbells into the air and then bring them together so they gently kiss. Bring them back down so your elbows and arms are at 90 degrees once again.

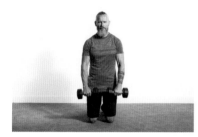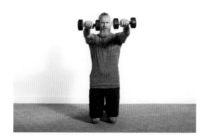

Transition into forward raises. Hold the dumbbells so they are touching your thighs and then lift both dumbbells up together with a slightly bent elbow to shoulder height and return to the start position.

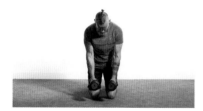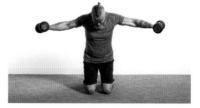

Transition into a bent-over row. Maintain a neutral spine, back and neck. The dumbbells are dangling in front of you beneath your chest and by your knees. With a slight bend in your elbows, retract the dumbbells so they are level with your shoulders and then return to the start position.

EXERCISE 3: ARMS MATRIX ON YOUR KNEES

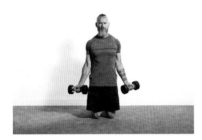 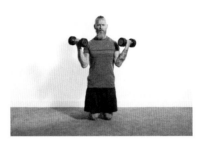 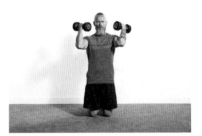

You're kneeling, which isolates the muscles. Hold a dumbbell in each hand so they are about 6 inches or 15 centimetres away from your legs, with your palms facing away from your body. Slowly raise your dumbbells up to shoulder height. Lift your elbows a couple of inches or 5 centimetres higher for extra pressure and then return to the start position.

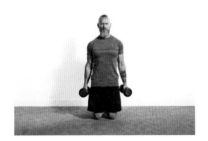 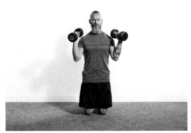 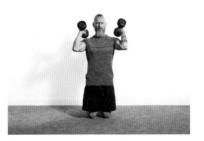

Change the hand position so your palms are now facing your body and the dumbbells are close to your legs. Curl the dumbbells up to shoulder height and then, with a little tip of the elbows which applies extra pressure on the bicep, return to the start position.

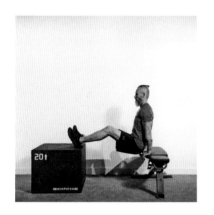 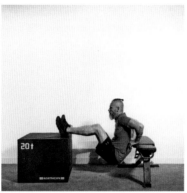

You'll need a bench for the tricep dips. For added resistance, use two benches and raise your legs. You should almost be sitting on your hands, with your fingers coming off the edge of the bench. Lower yourself down until your elbows are at 90 degrees. Return to the start position.

USING YOUR OWN BODYWEIGHT IS PHYSICALLY TOUGH BUT MENTALLY REWARDING.

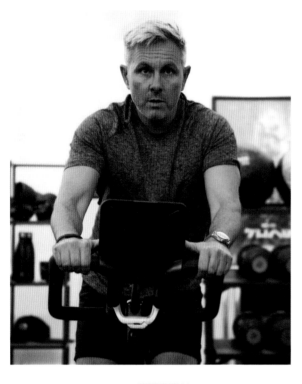
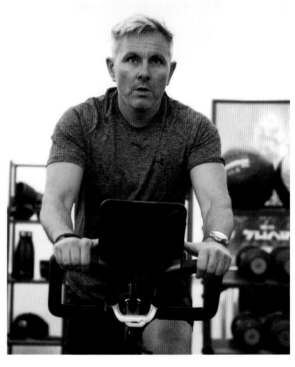
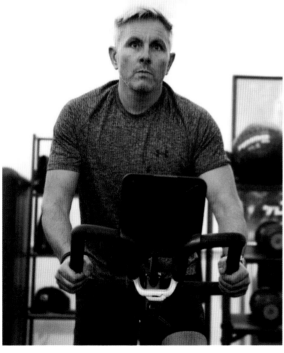
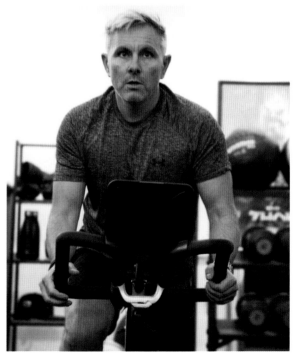

EXERCISE 4: DOUBLE DUMBBELL PLYOMETRIC

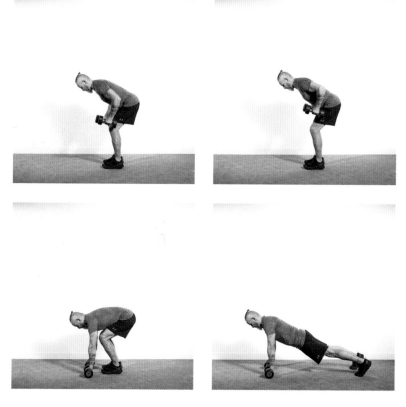

Holding two dumbbells, bend down into a squat position with your knees slightly soft and the weights around knee level. Bring both dumbbells into your chest and return to the start position. Put the weights on the ground and do the pylometric, with your legs shooting back and then forward. Return to the start position.

EXERCISE 5: CLEAN AND PRESS WITH DUMBBELLS (SEE PAGE 140)

DYNAMIC STRETCHING

▉	10–15 REPS / 20–30 SECONDS
▉	15–20 REPS / 30–40 SECONDS
▉	20–25 REPS / 40–50 SECONDS

EXERCISE 1: REVERSE LUNGE WITH A HIP-FLEXOR STRETCH

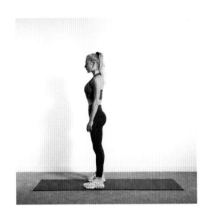 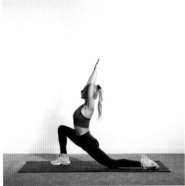

You're standing with your feet shoulder-width apart. Now step back and lower one knee to the ground. Your fingers are interlocked as you raise your hands above your head and lean back slightly, stretching your hip flexor. You can make this more dynamic by adding a forwards and backwards motion. Return to the start position and repeat with the other leg.

EXERCISE 2: QUAD-STRETCH REVERSE-LUNGE KNEE PULL

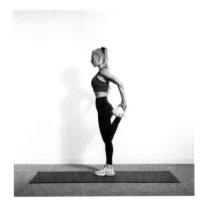 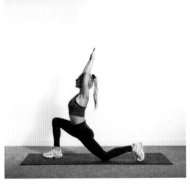 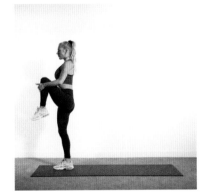

From a standing position, raise one leg behind you in a normal quad stretch, gripping the front of your foot. Hold for thirty seconds and then allow that leg to go backwards into a reverse lunge, with the knee touching the floor and arms locked above your head. Return to the start position, raising your knee in front of you, clasping it with both hands and then pulling it in tight. Now repeat with the other leg.

EXERCISE 3: PEDAL TO STANDING

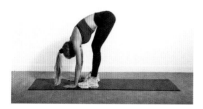 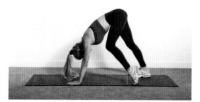

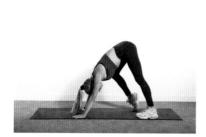 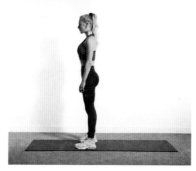

Start in the pike position, with your hands flat on the ground and your bottom in the air. Pedal your feet – left, right, left, right – so you always have one heel in the air. Walk that pedal forwards until your feet are between your hands, and then stand up slowly.

EXERCISE 4: UPPER-BODY MATRIX

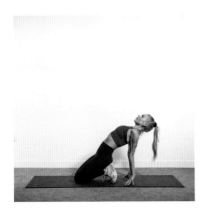
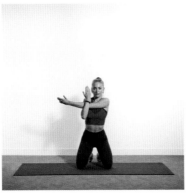

Kneel down and sit on your heels, with your hands behind you on the ground, stretching your shoulder and abdominal muscles. For the next stretch, maintain that kneeling position while bringing one arm across your body and hold it in place with the other. Pull your arm into your chest until you feel a comfortable stretch. Do the same with the other arm.

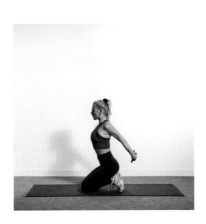
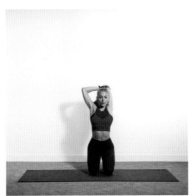

Now place your arms behind your back and clasp your hands together. Raise your hands slightly, bringing them up and away from your body, pushing your chest out slightly. Next move one arm up over your head and down your back, with your fingers pointing directly down your spine. Using your other hand, put a little bit of pressure on your elbow to stretch your triceps. Now do the same with the other arm.

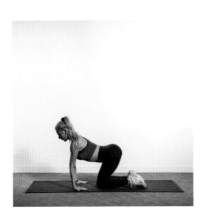
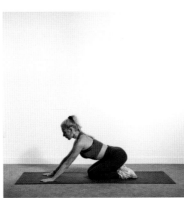

Then, place your palms on the floor, twisted so your fingers are pointing back towards you. You're stretching your forearm and leaning back slightly. Sit up and put your hands the other way around, with your fingers pointing in front of you. Rotate the wrists clockwise and then anticlockwise.

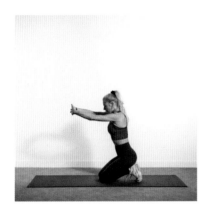 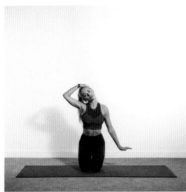

Now clasp your hands together and push them away from you, with your shoulder blades open. Hold and then return to the start position. Finish by putting your hand over your head with your fingers touching the opposite side. You're applying enough pressure so the head drops to one side, giving yourself a comfortable neck stretch. Do the same with your other arm.

EXERCISE 5: ABDUCTOR AND HAMSTRING MATRIX

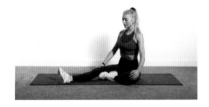 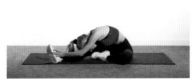 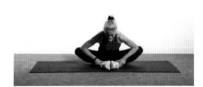

Sit up straight on the floor, with one leg straight out in front of you and the other leg pulled in with your heel on the inside of the first leg. Stretch up and out, reaching for your toes. Still sitting, bring the soles of your feet together and hold your ankles. Place your elbows on your knees and push down.

CORE

EXERCISE 1: BOSU ALTERNATE KNEE DRIVES

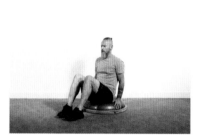 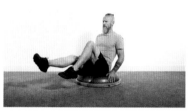 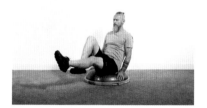

Sit on the BOSU hard side down, leaning back a little with your hands resting either side of it. Bring one knee up towards your chest, then lower it, and then do the same with the other knee, alternating between the legs. Once you've raised both knees, you've done one rep.

EXERCISE 2: BOSU LEG RAISES

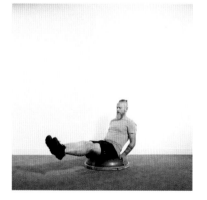 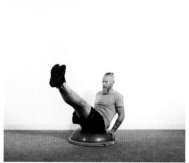

Sit on the BOSU, leaning back a little with your hands either side and with your legs raised parallel to the floor. Raise your legs to about 45 degrees, then return them to the start position. Keep your abdominals tight and engaged.

EXERCISE 3: BOSU HEEL TAPS

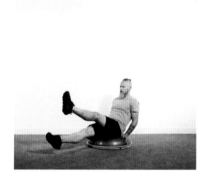 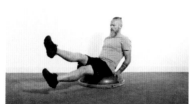

Sit on the BOSU, leaning back with your hands either side. Lift both legs off the ground at 90 degrees, keeping them straight. Touch one heel on the floor, then the other.

EXERCISE 4: MEDICINE BALL TWISTS

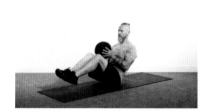 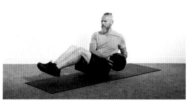 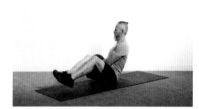

Sitting on the floor, with your feet slightly raised off the ground, hold a medicine ball, or any kind of weighted ball, in front of you. Rotate and touch the ball on the ground to your left. Return to the middle. Rotate and touch the ball on the ground on your right. Return to the middle.

EXERCISE 5: BOSU PLANK

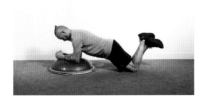 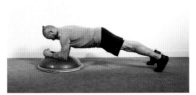

With your knees on the floor and your ankles crossed behind you, place your elbows on the BOSU and clasp your hands in front of you. Maintaining a tight core and glutes, hold this position for a set amount of time depending on your progress (see reps guide). For an advanced version of this, keep your hips and knees raised in the plank position instead.

ALWAYS KEEP YOUR GOAL IN MIND – NEVER LOSE SIGHT OF THAT.

CORE VARIETY FOR WEEKS 7–9

Depending on which equipment you have access to, you might wish to add some variety. Here are a few options for you to try.

CAGE CRUNCHES

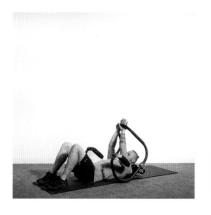 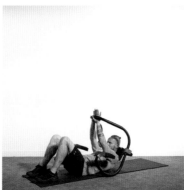

Lie on the floor with light fingers on the cage and your head resting on the pad. Raise yourself, squeeze the abs and then lower yourself down. You might find that using a cage gives you more control throughout the movement.

If you don't have access to a cage, you can control your tempo on these crunches by counting 3 seconds up and 3 seconds down.

CAGE CRUNCHES WITH RAISED KNEES

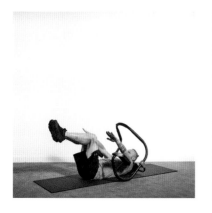 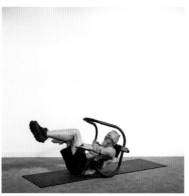

Lie on the floor with your head resting on the pad. Bring your knees up towards your chest while keeping your upper torso linear and applying pressure on the cage with your forearms. Raise yourself up, squeezing the abs while bringing both knees in at the same time. Return to the start position.

AROUND-THE-WORLD KETTLEBELL SWINGS

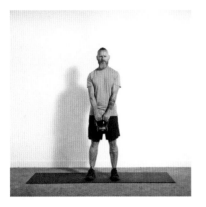
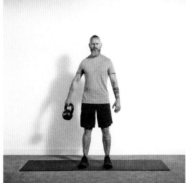

With slightly soft knees and your abs engaged, pick up a kettlebell. Pass the kettlebell around your body, clockwise from front to back, from one hand to the other. As you're off balance because of the weights, you're having to stabilize yourself through your core with this exercise.

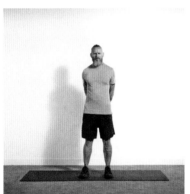
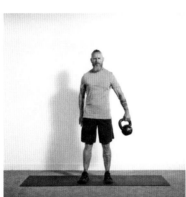

YOUR BODY DOESN'T JUST MOVE FORWARDS AND BACKWARDS AND FROM SIDE TO SIDE – IT ALSO LIKES TO ROTATE. THAT WILL IMPROVE YOUR DYNAMIC FLEXIBILITY.

SWISS BALL V-SIT

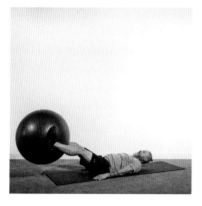 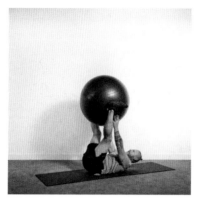 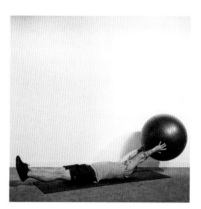

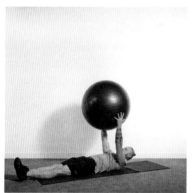 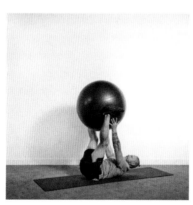

Lying on the floor, place a Swiss ball on the ground between your feet. Grasping the ball with both feet, raise your legs and grab the ball with your hands. Move your hands back until the Swiss ball touches the ground behind your head. Next, bring the ball back into the middle of your body. Move your feet up and clasp the ball with your feet. That's one rep.

AROUND-THE-WORLD SWISS BALL ROTATIONS

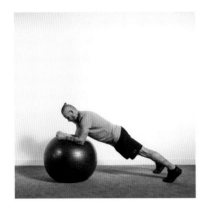 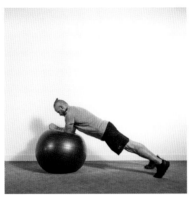

With your forearms resting on a Swiss ball, assume a plank position, with your legs straight out behind you. Push the ball away slightly so that your abs are engaged and your back is neutral. Roll your arms clockwise and then anticlockwise on the ball.

SWISS BALL ABDOMINAL ROPE PULL

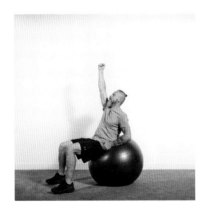 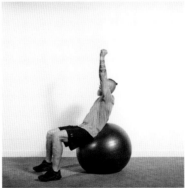

Sitting on a Swiss ball, with your feet on the floor, lean back and imagine you're pulling down on a rope with alternate hands while raising your upper body and crunching upwards.

FULL BODY

10–15 REPS / 20–30 SECONDS	
15–20 REPS / 30–40 SECONDS	
20–25 REPS / 40–50 SECONDS	

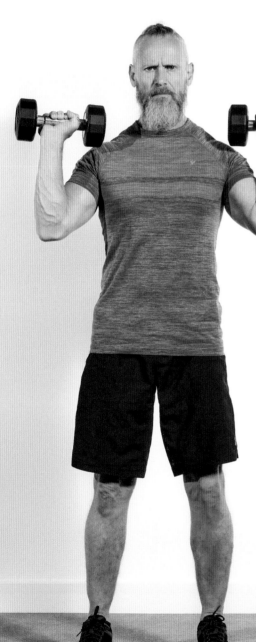

Exercise 1: Your weakest legs exercise

Exercise 2: Switch hand push-up with a knee drive
(see page 153)

Exercise 3: Weighted side lunge with a knee drive
(see page 150)

Exercise 4: Double dumbbell plyometric (see page 159)

Exercise 5: Clean and press with dumbbells (see page 140)

WEEK 7 RECAP

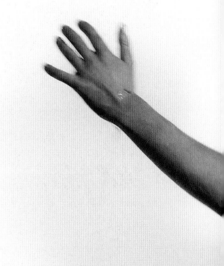

NUTRITION

○ Always have water with you throughout the day, and drink regularly. Sipping small amounts every so often is better than downing a huge amount in one go.

○ Gut health is very important, as that allows for good absorption and distribution, helping you to repair and giving you energy. To improve your gut health, you need probiotics, which we get from things like kimchi (fermented vegetables) or kefir (a fermented yoghurt). If you feel as though you have energy and you're sleeping well, that's often a sign that you have good gut health.

○ Don't be too purist about what you eat and have the same thing three times a day, seven days a week. If you stop eating certain food groups, your body might think it need not produce certain bacteria in your gut.

○ Keep learning about nutrition. Read as much as you can about what foods do for you and about portion sizes. Education goes a long way when it comes to nutrition.

WELLBEING

○ Your programme should help to give you a zest for life. The best compliment you can ever receive isn't about how you look, but that you're positive and full of energy.

○ If you weren't able to train at full intensity this week, don't beat yourself up. Remember that something is always better than nothing.

○ Go easy on yourself if something in your personal life is affecting your motivation to train. Do what you can today and fully engage tomorrow.

ACCUMULATOR: 5–4

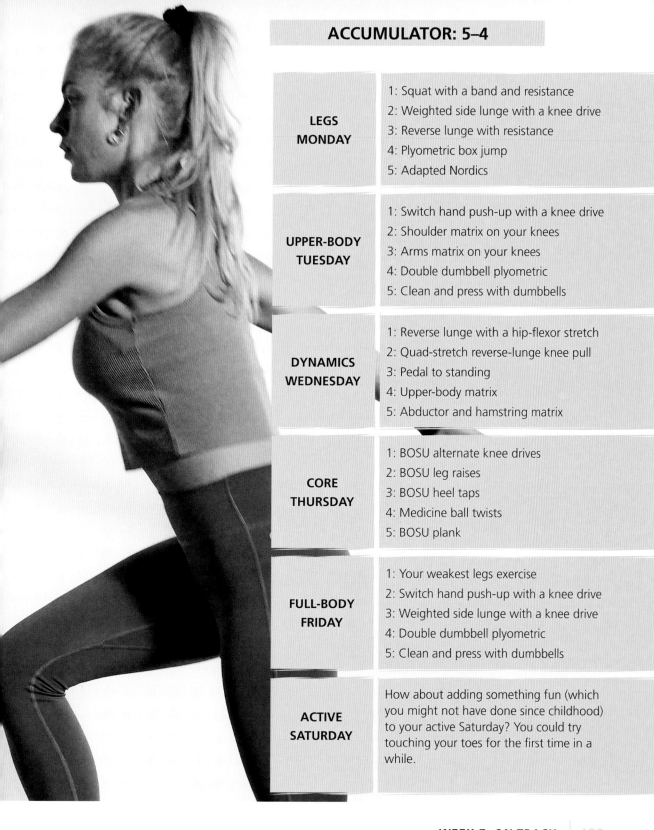

LEGS MONDAY	1: Squat with a band and resistance 2: Weighted side lunge with a knee drive 3: Reverse lunge with resistance 4: Plyometric box jump 5: Adapted Nordics
UPPER-BODY TUESDAY	1: Switch hand push-up with a knee drive 2: Shoulder matrix on your knees 3: Arms matrix on your knees 4: Double dumbbell plyometric 5: Clean and press with dumbbells
DYNAMICS WEDNESDAY	1: Reverse lunge with a hip-flexor stretch 2: Quad-stretch reverse-lunge knee pull 3: Pedal to standing 4: Upper-body matrix 5: Abductor and hamstring matrix
CORE THURSDAY	1: BOSU alternate knee drives 2: BOSU leg raises 3: BOSU heel taps 4: Medicine ball twists 5: BOSU plank
FULL-BODY FRIDAY	1: Your weakest legs exercise 2: Switch hand push-up with a knee drive 3: Weighted side lunge with a knee drive 4: Double dumbbell plyometric 5: Clean and press with dumbbells
ACTIVE SATURDAY	How about adding something fun (which you might not have done since childhood) to your active Saturday? You could try touching your toes for the first time in a while.

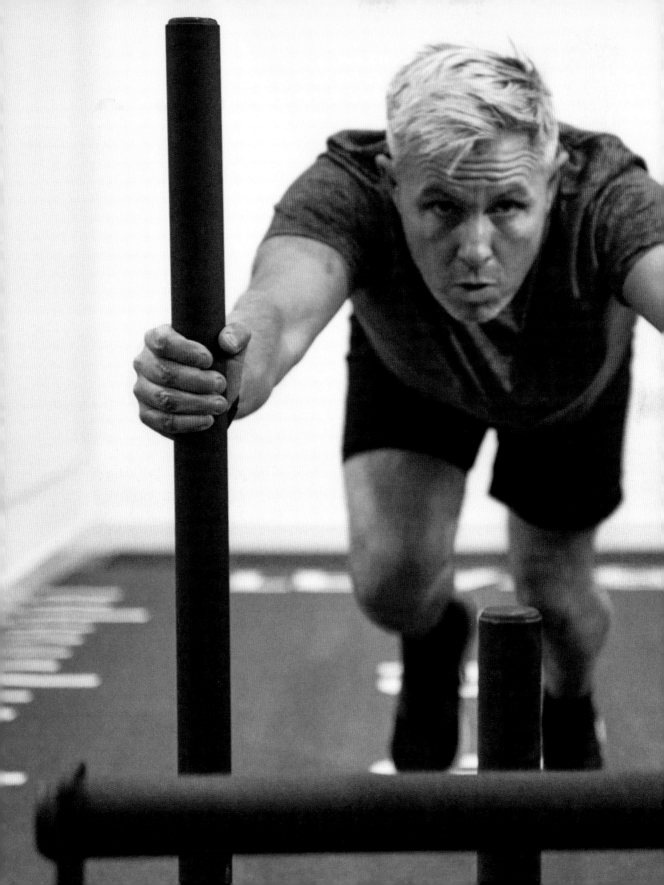

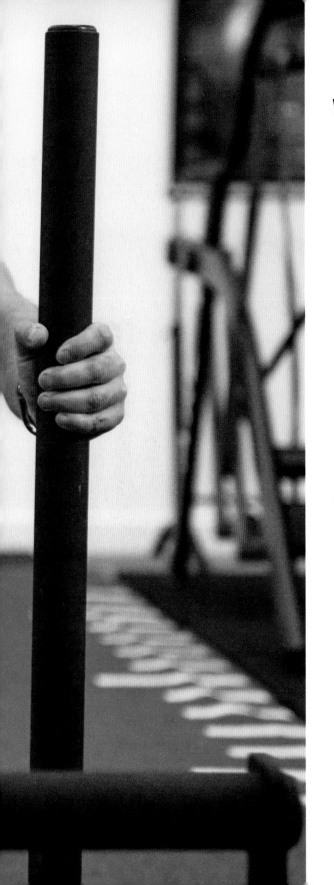

WEEK 8

'THE PREPARATION
TRAINING WITH SIMON
IS ESSENTIAL FOR ME.
FILMING A MOVIE
IS LIKE RUNNING A
MARATHON – IF YOU
DON'T ARRIVE WELL
PREPARED, YOU WILL
PAY FOR IT AT THE END.'
Diego Luna

ENJOY THE FEELING

As soon as you start to see results, your natural reaction is to want to do more, push even harder, as your end goal feels so close. We often think that more is more. But with fitness, that's not always the case. Less is often more.

ACCUMULATOR: 5–4

This is the point of the process where you might find yourself craving more sessions. Maybe just a couple of weeks ago, during the dreaded Week 6, you were thinking, 'I don't want to do anything,' but now you can't get enough. You always want to do something and perhaps you're thinking that you should do more. While it's fantastic to be motivated – and this is the time when you can make significant progress – be careful that you don't push too hard. Try to stay within the parameters I've given you.

I've had to restrain actors who want to work out more and more. However, in my experience, you can spend more time in the gym but not get the additional benefit from doing that. You could be asking too much of your body, and not be giving your muscles enough time to recover before you go again. If you're training at the right level, your body will be able to flush out the lactic acid and other toxins it produces after exercise. But if you're working beyond your capabilities, your body will take longer to get rid of the toxins and acids, and those chemicals will then sit in your muscle tissue, leading to soreness.

STAY ON THE PATH

If you're training more but you don't get the results you had been expecting, that can be disheartening and could actually affect your motivation. It can often be more effective to stay on the path or trajectory you're on, just incrementally increasing what you're doing (as you have been so far during this challenge). If your steady approach is working, and you're getting the results, stay with it. If you stick with the programme I have created, based on more than twenty-five years' experience and results, you may find that the sessions are a little easier and you feel fitter. That's a great feeling to have – enjoy it!

If you want to increase what you're doing, with greater resistance, additional reps or more intense cardio, still do 10 or 20 per cent less than what you imagine you're capable of. That will make it more sustainable and will allow you to keep going for the rest of the challenge – and beyond. Another reason not to do too much this week is that next week is when you get to test your limits. You'll want to be in the best possible state for that. Take any additional energy you have this week and inject that into other parts of your life, such as your work or family. Enjoy that feeling, that energy boost.

PURE STRENGTH OR PURE CARDIO

To mix it up, I'm giving you the option of doing a 'pure strength' or a 'pure cardio' week, depending on what your goals are, though you're still using the same methodology that you have throughout with my trusted accumulator. For a pure strength week, you can replace the cardio element of your workouts with the core exercises I have given you for Thursday. If you like the idea of a pure cardio week, the cardio element should be more dynamic. That could mean ladder work, which is all about freestyling and having lots of variety. Use the ladder as a tool to be creative, with linear work, lateral work, and steps, jumps and bounds. You could also

WEEK 8 KIT LIST

ANKLE WEIGHTS
BAR AND WEIGHTS
BENCH
BOSU
BOX
DUMBBELLS
SWISS BALL

OPTIONAL
(for core variety)
CAGE
KETTLEBELL
SWISS BALL

try being creative with the BOSU, with the soft side up, to build speed, agility and diversity. Or you could do plyometrics for your cardio. Where possible, swap any exercises using resistance for ones that are more movement-based. But don't feel the need to change it up: you might want to stick to what you have been doing.

On Thursday, please don't forget that you have a greater choice of core exercises (see Week 7 for the step-by-step instructions on how to do those correctly and safely).

LEGS

EXERCISE 1: SWISS BALL SQUAT

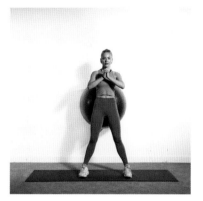 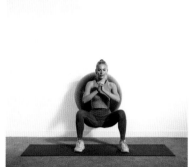

Hold a Swiss ball against the wall with the middle of your back, with your feet shoulder-width apart and your toes pointing slightly outwards. Your arms can be dangling by your sides or you can clasp your hands in front of you with your elbows high, which helps to give you a neutral spine. Slide down the wall until the Swiss ball is at your upper back and, with your legs at 90 degrees, hold that position for a count of four. Explode through your heels to return to the start position.

BEING FIT IS A GREAT FEELING. SAVOUR THAT.

EXERCISE 2: WEIGHTED SIDE LUNGE WITH A KNEE DRIVE AND ANKLE WEIGHTS

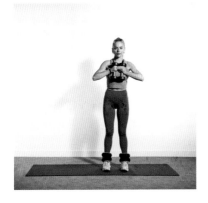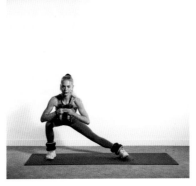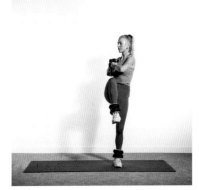

Wearing ankle weights for extra resistance, hold moderate weights in front of you in the middle of your chest. Take a step to your right and then go into a squat position on that side while keeping your left leg straight. Pushing through the heel, return to the start position and transition into a knee drive, with your right knee at 90 degrees out in front of you and your upper body twisted to the right. Return to the start position and repeat with the opposite leg.

EXERCISE 3: REVERSE LUNGE WITH A JUMP

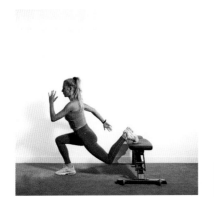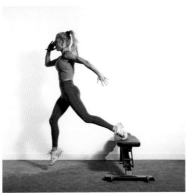

Stand with your feet shoulder-width apart and one foot on a bench behind you. Drop your back knee to the floor in a lunge position. Push upwards, returning to the start position, and then do a small jump in the air with your front foot. Do the reps and then switch legs.

EXERCISE 4: PLYOMETRIC BOX JUMP WITH RESISTANCE

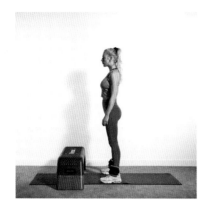 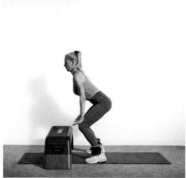 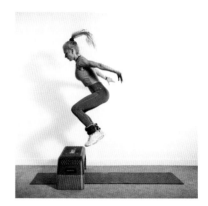

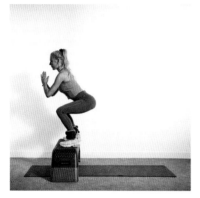 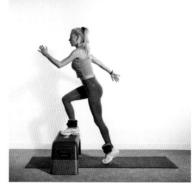 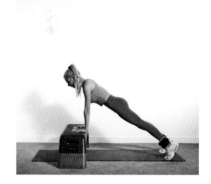

Wearing ankle weights, stand 10 inches or 25 centimetres back from the box with your feet shoulder-width apart and your arms by your sides. Get into a squat position. Propel yourself through the air, landing with both feet on the box. Step down from the box. Now put your hands on the box and shoot your legs back and then forwards. Return to the start position.

EXERCISE 5: ADAPTED NORDICS (SEE PAGE 152)

UPPER BODY

	10–15 REPS / 20–30 SECONDS
	15–20 REPS / 30–40 SECONDS
	20–25 REPS / 40–50 SECONDS

EXERCISE 1: PUSH-UP WITH A SIDE KNEE DRIVE

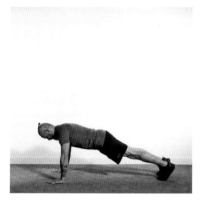 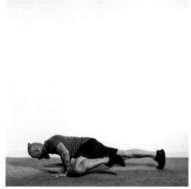

Place your hands on the ground shoulder-width apart. Lower yourself down until your elbows are at 90 degrees, driving one knee up to the side of your elbow. Push up and return to the start position, breathing out on exertion. Now do the same with the other leg, alternating between the two.

TRY NOT TO FORCE IT OR PUSH TOO HARD NOW, AS THAT COULD JEOPARDIZE THE REST OF THE CHALLENGE.

EXERCISE 2: SHOULDER MATRIX ON YOUR KNEES WITH A SLOW TEMPO

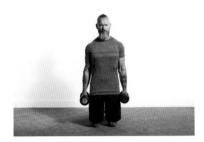 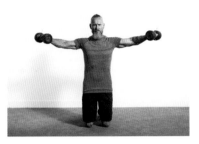

In a kneeling position, you can't use your legs and you're isolating the upper body. By slowing down the tempo of the exercise, you're increasing the time that your muscles are under tension. For the lateral raises, slowly lift the dumbbells to the side with slightly bent elbows so they are level with your shoulders. Return to the start position.

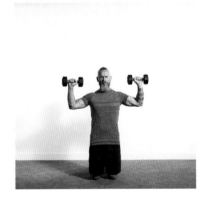 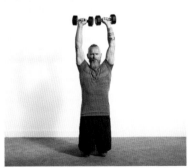

Transition from lateral raises into a shoulder press. Hold the dumbbells so that your arms are at 90 degrees on either side and the dumbbells are about 6 inches or 15 centimetres away from your ears. Raise the dumbbells slowly into the air and then bring them together so they gently kiss. Bring them back down so your elbows and arms are at 90 degrees once again.

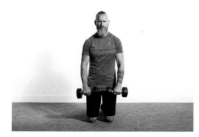 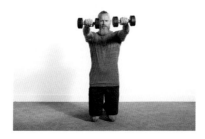

Transition into forward raises. Hold the dumbbells so they are touching your thighs and then slowly lift both dumbbells up with a slightly bent elbow to shoulder height and return to the start position.

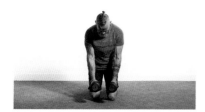 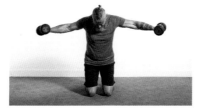

Transition into a bent-over row. Maintaining a neutral spine, back and neck, hold the dumbbells in front of you beneath the chest and by your knees. With a slight bend in your elbows, slowly retract the dumbbells so they are level with your shoulders and then return to the start position.

EXERCISE 3: ARMS MATRIX ON YOUR KNEES (SEE PAGE 156)

EXERCISE 4: DOUBLE DUMBBELL PLYOMETRIC AND PUSH-UP

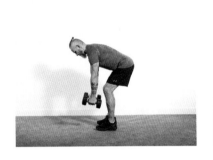 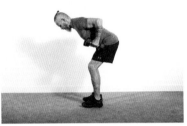 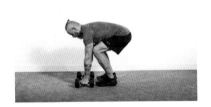

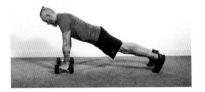 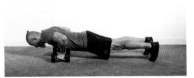

Holding two dumbbells, bend down into the squat position with your knees slightly soft. The weights should be halfway between your knees and ankles. Pull the dumbbells into your chest and then return to the start position.

Now put the weights on the ground and do the plyometric, with your legs shooting back. Do a push up, and then jump your legs back towards the dumbbells before returning to the start position.

EXERCISE 5: CLEAN AND PRESS WITH A PLYOMETRIC

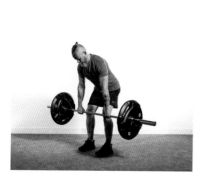 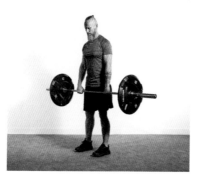 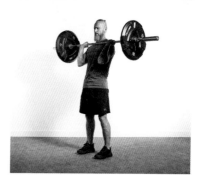

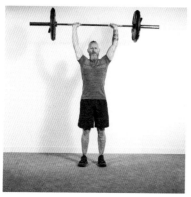 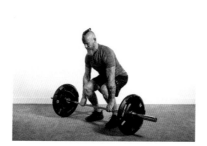 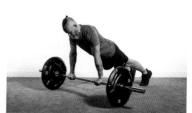

Put a moderate weight on the bar and stand in front of it, feet shoulder-width apart. Use an overhand grip, and keep a neutral back and neck. As you lift the bar up, it will naturally brush your thighs. With your elbows high, flip the bar over so that your palms are facing the ceiling. Raise the bar until your elbows are locked out or straight. Return the bar to your chest and allow it to flip back to your thighs and back down to the ground. Stand with your feet shoulder-width apart and then squat down. Shoot your legs out together behind you and then bring them back towards the bar before returning to the start position. Keep hold of the bar at all times.

DYNAMIC STRETCHING

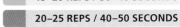

10–15 REPS / 20–30 SECONDS	
15–20 REPS / 30–40 SECONDS	
20–25 REPS / 40–50 SECONDS	

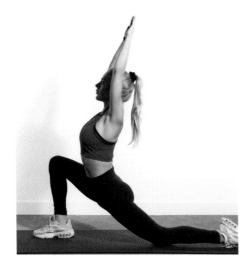

Exercise 1: Reverse lunge with a hip-flexor stretch
(see page 160)

Exercise 2: Quad-stretch reverse-lunge knee pull
(see page 160)

Exercise 3: Pedal to standing (see page 161)

Exercise 4: Upper-body matrix (see page 162)

Exercise 5: Abductor and hamstring matrix (see page 163)

CORE

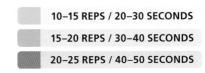

10–15 REPS / 20–30 SECONDS	
15–20 REPS / 30–40 SECONDS	
20–25 REPS / 40–50 SECONDS	

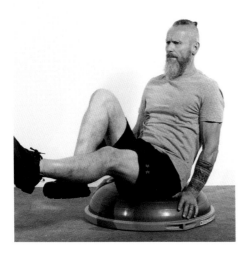

Exercise 1: BOSU alternate knee drives (see page 164)

Exercise 2: BOSU leg raises (see page 164)

Exercise 3: BOSU heel taps (see page 165)

Exercise 4: Medicine ball twists (see page 165)

Exercise 5: BOSU plank (see page 166)

FULL BODY

Exercise 1: Your weakest legs exercise
Exercise 2: Push-up with a side knee drive (see page 181)
Exercise 3: Weighted side lunge with a knee drive and
ankle weights (see page 179)
Exercise 4: Double dumbbell plyometric and push-up
(see page 184)
Exercise 5: Clean and press with a plyometric (see page 185)

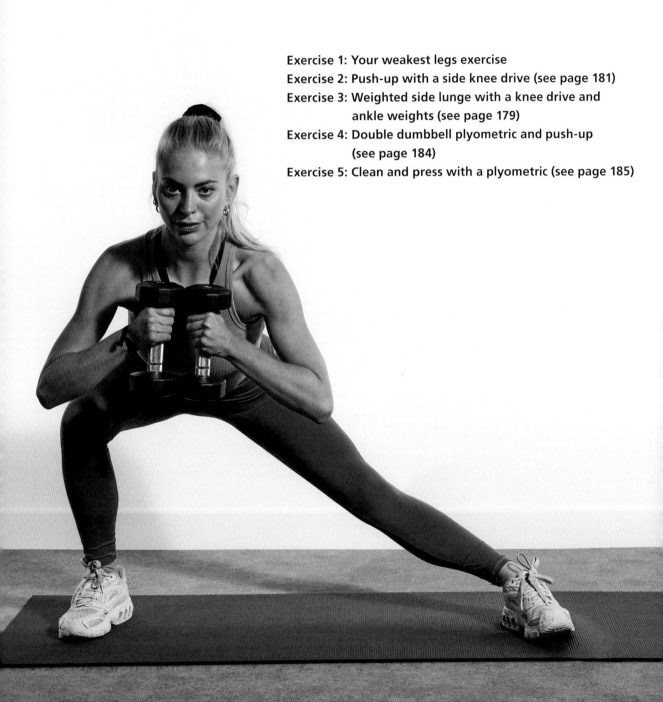

WEEK 8 RECAP

NUTRITION

○ I like theme days because they help you to set parameters for your nutrition without being too restrictive or boring. You could think about Vegetarian Mondays, Pescatarian Tuesdays, Vegan Wednesdays, White Meat Thursdays and Red Meat Fridays. But see what suits you and what's going to be sustainable. Feel free to change the theme if you're out for lunch or dinner and it's simply not going to be possible to stick to it that day.

○ Don't be an antisocial butterfly. That means not imposing your nutritional plan on anyone else. Everyone is going to have a different relationship with food, and you don't want to be that nightmare dinner guest because you're so rigid with your diet! Don't stress about taking an evening out from your eating plan.

WELLBEING

○ Remember that if you don't allow yourself to recover, you're not going to make progress in this programme. Take your recovery as seriously as your workouts.

○ Swimming in cold water will boost your immune system and also help to flush the toxins out of your body. Being in water is also great for recovery as it takes much of your weight, reducing the strain on your body.

○ Sleep is the most important recovery tool. If you're getting good sleep, you should be recovering well.

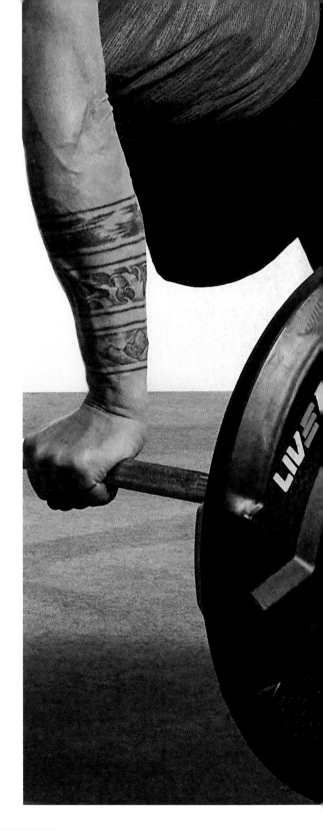

LEGS MONDAY	1: Swiss ball squat 2: Weighted side lunge with a knee drive and ankle weights 3: Reverse lunge with a jump 4: Plyometric box jump with resistance 5: Adapted Nordics
UPPER-BODY TUESDAY	1: Push-up with a side knee drive 2: Shoulder matrix on your knees with a slow tempo 3: Arms matrix on your knees 4: Double dumbbell plyometric and push-up 5: Clean and press with a plyometric
DYNAMICS WEDNESDAY	1: Reverse lunge with a hip-flexor stretch 2: Quad-stretch reverse-lunge knee pull 3: Pedal to standing 4: Upper-body matrix 5: Abductor and hamstring matrix
CORE THURSDAY	1: BOSU alternate knee drives 2: BOSU leg raises 3: BOSU heel taps 4: Medicine ball twists 5: BOSU plank
FULL-BODY FRIDAY	1: Your weakest legs exercise 2: Push-up with a side knee drive 3: Weighted side lunge with a knee drive and ankle weights 4: Double dumbbell plyometric and push-up 5: Clean and press with a plyometric
ACTIVE SATURDAY	If you respond well to a competitive element, maybe there's a challenge you could do with a friend or family member. It could be your own mini-triathlon or something simpler.

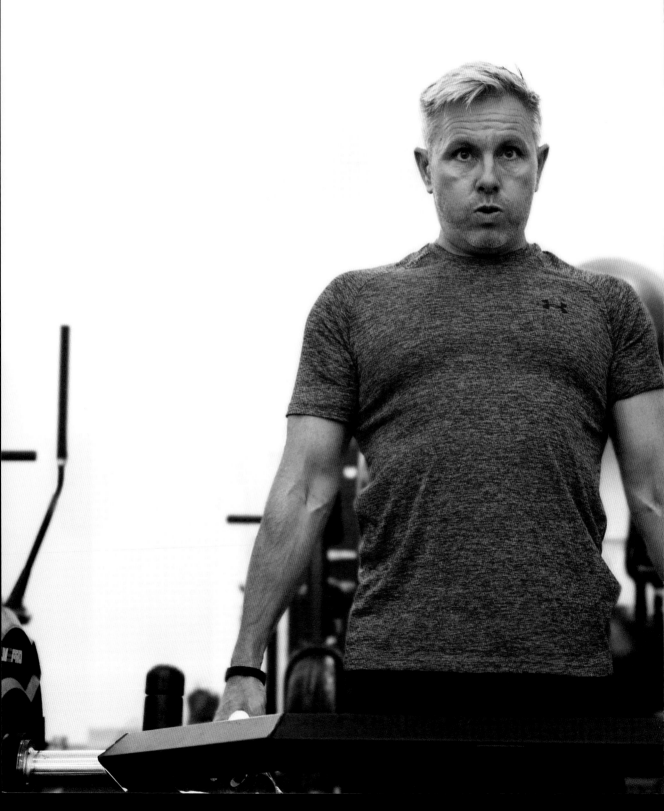

WEEK 9

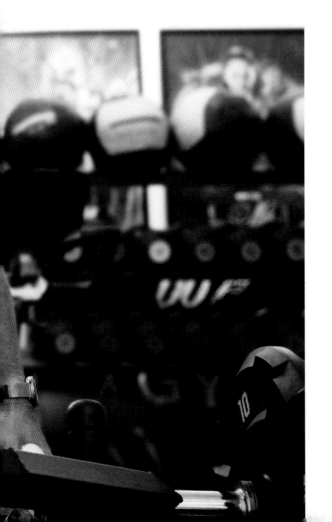

'SIMON DOESN'T JUST HELP YOU TO ENHANCE YOUR PHYSICAL CAPABILITIES – HE ALSO ENSURES YOU WALK OUT OF THE GYM FEELING AMAZING ABOUT YOURSELF.'
Luke Evans

TEST YOUR LIMITS

This week is the absolute pinnacle. This is when you'll be testing yourself to see how far you can go. It's the week when you find out where your limits are.

ACCUMULATOR: 5–5

You're controlling how you move your body, how you rest it and how you fuel it. This is the moment in the programme when I like to tell clients who are fitter, stronger and more resilient than ever before: 'You're in control now.' So now that you're fully in charge, what are you going to do with your new capability? This week you get the chance to move your body as you wish. Week 9 can be brutal if you want it to be – it's all about testing your new limits.

Perhaps you think that I've been holding you back over the past couple of weeks and you could have gone a bit further. This is your chance to challenge yourself and go beyond what you have done so far in this programme. If you want this week to be intense, go ahead and do it, as I think you're capable. That could mean more reps, moving up from beginner to intermediate or from intermediate to advanced, or trying out slightly heavier weights.

But this isn't an invitation to be reckless. Always make sure you're testing yourself safely. You don't want to hurt yourself right at the end of this programme as this is a time to be feeling good about your progress and what you're capable of, rather than sustaining an injury. Make sure that everything is achievable and that you're not asking too much of yourself. I wouldn't, for instance, recommend going from beginner to advanced in the space of a week.

SEE WHERE YOU CAN TAKE IT

When you're testing your limits, be a little flexible and carefree with your approach. Tell yourself you'll see where it goes and where you can take it. Don't start having delusions about what you can accomplish – you probably won't suddenly be able to do fifty push-ups. Avoid setting yourself overly ambitious targets that you're almost certain to fail.

IS THAT ALL YOU'VE GOT?

When you think you've reached your limit on a particular exercise, sit down, think, rest and pause for ten seconds and then return to it straightaway. Don't be afraid to coach yourself, asking yourself how far you can go this week, and motivate yourself to push a little bit harder. That's something I've often done in the past when I've been training, asking myself: 'Simon, is that all you've got?' I find that often works; you usually have a little more you can give.

Be creative this week. Maybe put on some ankle weights or a weighted jacket when working out. This week is a chance to try something different and to take it somewhere fresh. You might want to do different cardio. Perhaps you've been on the exercise bike for all your cardio throughout the challenge. Why don't you get on the treadmill this week and see what you're capable of? When you're doing your core workout on Thursday, please don't forget you have some choice (see Week 7 for the step-by-step instructions on how to do those exercises correctly and safely). For your active recovery on Saturday, why not try a new sport, and if you're planning on going for a walk on Sunday, you could look at exploring somewhere new that encourages you to walk that little bit further.

You will have noticed that I've increased the cardio this week to five minutes. I think you can handle that at this point in the programme. It's a total of twenty-five minutes of cardio for your daily session, which should be very achievable at this stage.

WEEK 9 KIT LIST

ANKLE WEIGHTS
BANDS
BAR AND WEIGHTS
BENCH
BOSU
BOX
DUMBBELLS
DUMBBELL, KETTLEBELL OR MEDICINE BALL
STEP
WEIGHTED JACKET

OPTIONAL (for core variety)
CAGE
KETTLEBELL
SWISS BALL

LEGS

10–15 REPS / 20–30 SECONDS	
15–20 REPS / 30–40 SECONDS	
20–25 REPS / 40–50 SECONDS	

EXERCISE 1: WIDE SQUAT WITH RESISTANCE

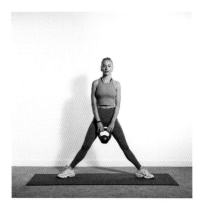 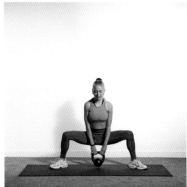

Hold a dumbbell, kettlebell or medicine ball with both hands between your legs, with your feet wider than shoulder-width apart and your toes pointing outwards. Lower yourself down until the resistance item touches the ground and your knees are at 90 degrees, then hold that position for a count of four. Explode through your heels to return to the start position.

EXERCISE 2: BALLISTIC BANDED WEIGHTED SQUATS

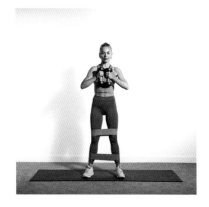 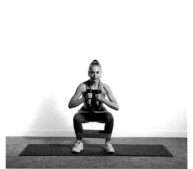 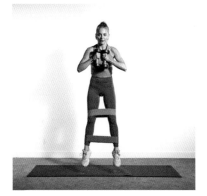

With one band above your ankles and another just above your knees, hold a pair of dumbbells against your chest. Squat down to 90 degrees, and as you reach the bottom, drive through your heels and jump about 6 inches or 15 centimetres into the air. Landing on your heels, go straight back into the squat.

EXERCISE 3: THREE-AND-THREE BALLISTIC LUNGE

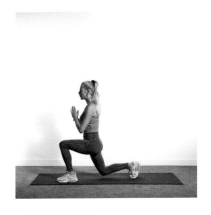
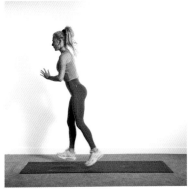

Stand with your feet shoulder-width apart. Lunge forward, dropping your rear leg until your knee kisses the floor. Power upwards, returning to the start position. Do three lunges on one side, then three skips, which means you'll be switching to the other leg. Now do three lunges on the other side and three skips. That's one rep.

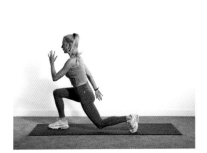
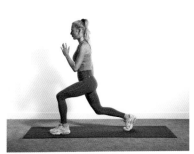

WHEN TESTING YOUR LIMITS, IT HELPS TO BE FLEXIBLE IN YOUR APPROACH. DON'T TRY TO GO BEYOND WHAT YOUR BODY IS CAPABLE OF.

EXERCISE 4: PLYOMETRIC BOX JUMP WITH RESISTANCE AND A SQUAT

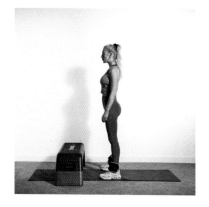 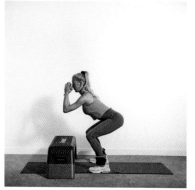 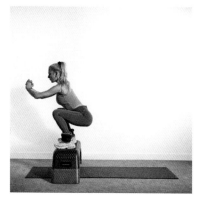

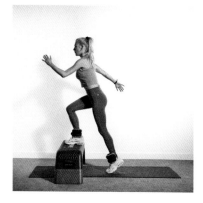 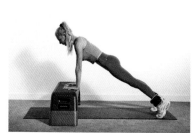

Wearing ankle weights, stand 10 inches or 25 centimetres back from the box with your feet shoulder-width apart and your arms by your sides. Get into a squat position. Propel yourself through the air. Land with both feet on the box. Do a squat on top of the box. Step down from the box. Put your hands on the box, shoot your legs back and then forwards, and return to the start position.

EXERCISE 5: ADAPTED NORDICS WITH A BOSU OR STEP PUSH-UP

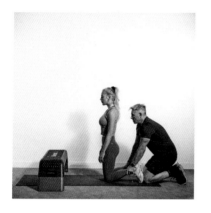 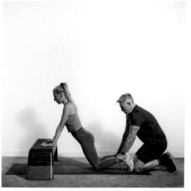 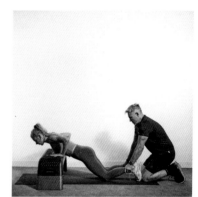

You're in a kneeling position but with your heels tucked under something, like a bench. If you have a training partner, ask them to hold your legs. You have a BOSU or step in front of you. Lower yourself down gradually, keeping your glutes and hamstrings tight, until your hands hit the BOSU or step. Lower yourself until your elbows are at 90 degrees. Push yourself up, returning to the start position.

YOUR MENTAL STRENGTH AND AGILITY SHOULD NOW MATCH YOUR PHYSICAL STRENGTH AND AGILITY.

UPPER BODY

	10–15 REPS / 20–30 SECONDS
	15–20 REPS / 30–40 SECONDS
	20–25 REPS / 40–50 SECONDS

EXERCISE 1: PUSH-UP WITH A KICK-THROUGH

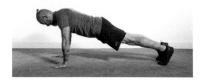 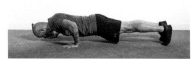 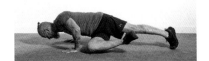

Place your hands on the ground shoulder-width apart with your legs straight behind you. If this exercise is new to you, you might find it easier to rest your knees on the ground and to cross your ankles behind you. Lower yourself down until your elbows are at 90 degrees. Push up and return to the start position, breathing out on exertion. Lower yourself down again and bring your right knee through towards the opposite arm. On the next rep, swap legs and bring the other knee through to the other arm.

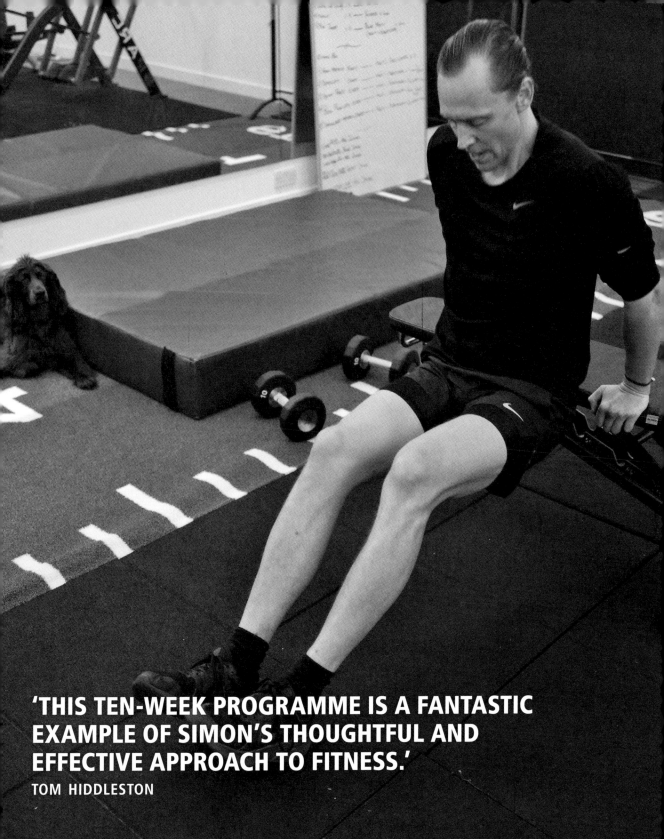

'THIS TEN-WEEK PROGRAMME IS A FANTASTIC EXAMPLE OF SIMON'S THOUGHTFUL AND EFFECTIVE APPROACH TO FITNESS.'
TOM HIDDLESTON

EXERCISE 2: SHOULDER MATRIX ON YOUR KNEES WITH HALF MOVEMENTS

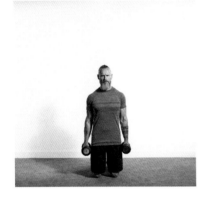 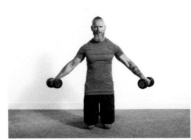

In a kneeling position, you can't use your legs and you're isolating the upper body. You're doing half movements for the lateral raises (and forward raises if you'd like a more intense exercise now), which means the muscles are under constant tension. For the lateral raises, lift the dumbbells to the side with slightly bent elbows so they are halfway to being level with your ears. Return to the start position.

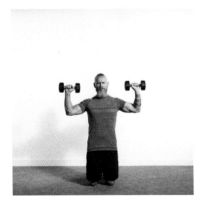 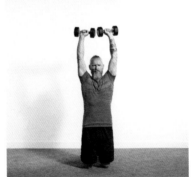

Transition from lateral raises into a shoulder press. Hold the dumbbells so that your arms are at 90 degrees on either side and the dumbbells are about 6 inches or 15 centimetres away from your ears. Raise the dumbbells into the air and then bring them together so they gently kiss. Bring them back down so your elbows and arms are at 90 degrees once again.

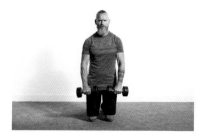
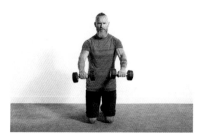

Transition into forward raises. Hold the dumbbells so they are touching your thighs and then lift both dumbbells up together with a slightly bent elbow, so they're at shoulder height (or halfway if you want to push it a little more), and return to the start position.

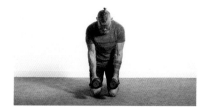
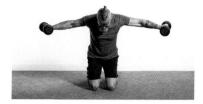

Transition into a bent-over row. Maintain a neutral spine, back and neck. The dumbbells are dangling in front of you beneath your chest and by your knees. With a slight bend in your elbows, retract the dumbbells so they are level with your shoulders and then return to the start position.

EXERCISE 3: ARMS MATRIX ON YOUR KNEES (SEE PAGE 156)

EXERCISE 4: BARBELL ROW INTO PLYOMETRIC AND PRESS-UP INTO ROLLOUT

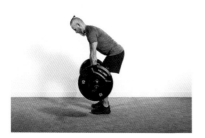 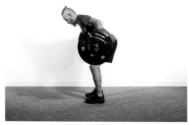 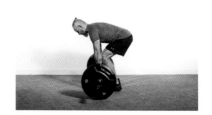

This is pretty challenging, and not for the faint-hearted. Please feel free to adapt this to your ability – you could always omit the rollout.

After adding the right amount of weights to suit your ability, place the bar in front of you. Bend your knees. Keeping a neutral back, use an overhand grip to clasp the bar and bring it up to your knees. Slide the bar up your thighs into your waist, retracting the back and squeezing the lats. Put the barbell on the ground.

For the plyometric, hold the barbell with both hands and shoot your legs back. Then do a press up before jumping your feet back towards the barbell.

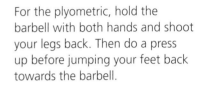

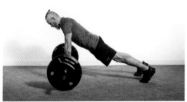

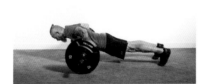

Next, drop onto your knees and push the barbell out in front of you, engaging your core while keeping your back neutral and flat. Bring the barbell back and return to the original standing position to lift the bar.

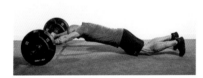

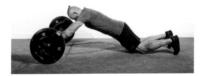

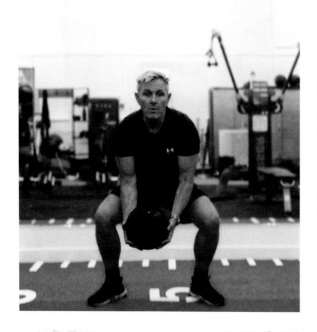
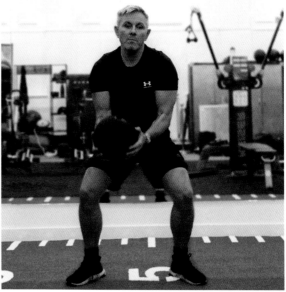
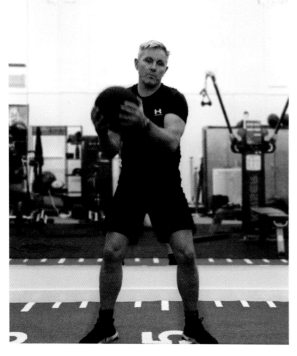
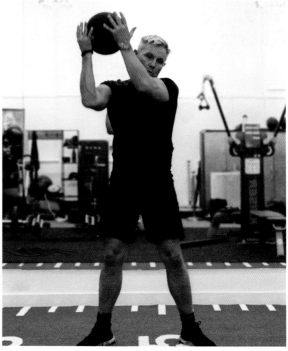

EXERCISE 5: CLEAN AND PRESS WITH A PLYOMETRIC AND A PUSH-UP

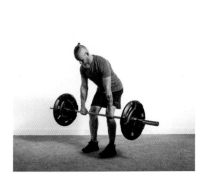
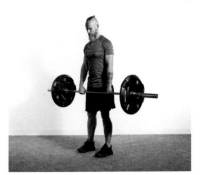
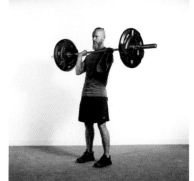

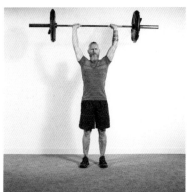
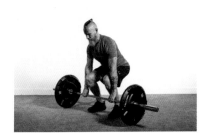
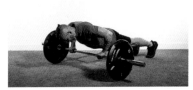

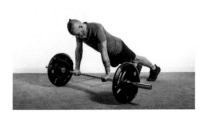

Put a moderate weight on the bar and stand in front of it with your feet shoulder-width apart. Use an overhand grip, and keep a neutral back and neck. As you lift the bar up, it will naturally brush your thighs. With your elbows high, flip the bar over so that your palms are facing the ceiling. Raise the bar until your elbows are locked out or straight. Return the bar to your chest and allow it to flip back to your thighs and back down to the ground.

Now squat down and shoot your legs out together behind you. Lower yourself down until your elbows are at 90 degrees. Do a push-up, jump your feet back towards the bar and return to the start position, breathing out on exertion.

DYNAMIC STRETCHING

	10–15 REPS / 20–30 SECONDS
	15–20 REPS / 30–40 SECONDS
	20–25 REPS / 40–50 SECONDS

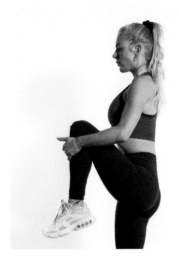

Exercise 1: Reverse lunge with a hip-flexor stretch
(see page 160)

Exercise 2: Quad-stretch reverse-lunge knee pull
(see page 160)

Exercise 3: Pedal to standing (see page 161)

Exercise 4: Upper-body matrix (see page 162)

Exercise 5: Abductor and hamstring matrix (see page 163)

WEEK 9 / **THURSDAY**

CORE

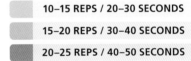

	10–15 REPS / 20–30 SECONDS
	15–20 REPS / 30–40 SECONDS
	20–25 REPS / 40–50 SECONDS

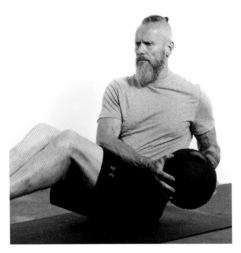

Exercise 1: BOSU alternate knee drives (see page 164)

Exercise 2: BOSU leg raises (see page 164)

Exercise 3: BOSU heel taps (see page 165)

Exercise 4: Medicine ball twists (see page 165)

Exercise 5: BOSU plank (see page 166)

FULL BODY

Exercise 1: Your weakest legs exercise
Exercise 2: Push-up with a kick-through (see page 198)
Exercise 3: Ballistic banded weighted squats (see page 194)
Exercise 4: Barbell row into plyometric and press-up into rollout (see page 202)
Exercise 5: Clean and press with a plyometric and a push-up (see page 205)

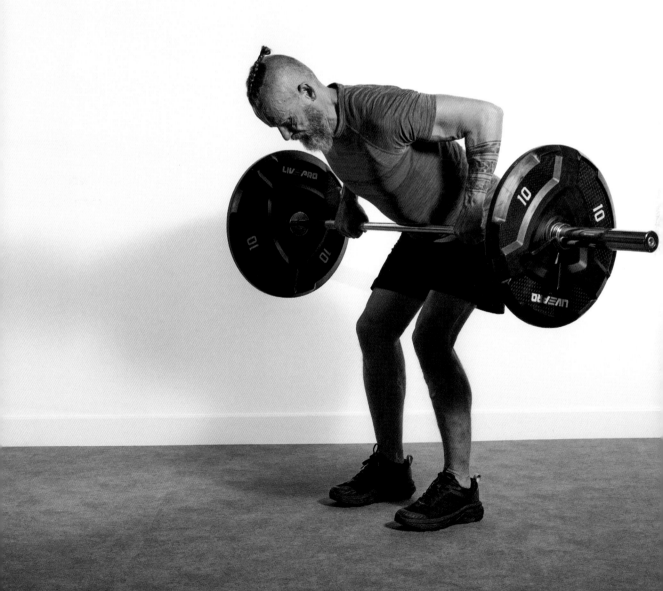

WEEK 9 RECAP

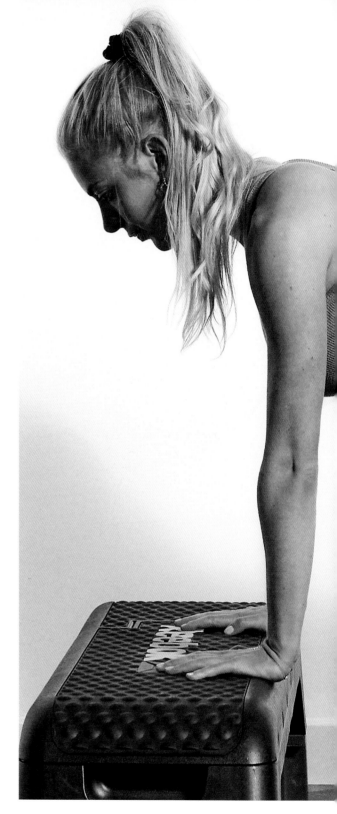

NUTRITION

○ As the intensity is at its highest this week, make sure you're consuming foods with anti-inflammatory properties. A daily ginger shot or a cup of turmeric tea will help to put your body into an anti-inflammatory state.

○ Ensure you're eating enough protein for muscle repair. And look into getting your protein from different sources.

○ I always think it's a bad idea to talk about a 'cheat' meal. Nothing's cheating. Don't put that label on what you eat.

WELLBEING

○ Extend your post-workout stretching routine.

○ For a restorative bath, add some Epsom salts to the water, which can help relax muscles and reduce swelling.

○ For cold-water therapy, which will aid your recovery, can you have a cold shower for a minute or two at the end of your hot shower? Focus on your breathing, which will help you to deal with the shock of the cold.

○ In the winter, when we don't get much sun, you could think about taking a vitamin D supplement. At any time of the year, you might want to consider a good multi-vitamin or multi-mineral supplement, and perhaps also a probiotic supplement and one for omega acids.

ACCUMULATOR: 5–5

LEGS MONDAY	1: Wide squat with resistance 2: Ballistic banded weighted squats 3: Three-and-three ballistic lunge 4: Plyometric box jump with resistance and a squat 5: Adapted Nordics with a BOSU or step push-up
UPPER-BODY TUESDAY	1: Push-up with a kick-through 2: Shoulder matrix on your knees with half movements 3: Arms matrix on your knees 4: Barbell row into plyometric and press-up into rollout 5: Clean and press with a plyometric and a push-up
DYNAMICS WEDNESDAY	1: Reverse lunge with a hip-flexor stretch 2: Quad-stretch reverse-lunge knee pull 3: Pedal to standing 4: Upper-body matrix 5: Abductor and hamstring matrix
CORE THURSDAY	1: BOSU alternate knee drives 2: BOSU leg raises 3: BOSU heel taps 4: Medicine ball twists 5: BOSU plank
FULL-BODY FRIDAY	1: Your weakest legs exercise 2: Push-up with a kick-through 3: Ballistic banded weighted squats 4: Barbell row into plyometric and press-up into rollout 5: Clean and press with a plyometric and a push-up
ACTIVE SATURDAY	Go for a long hike, maybe exploring somewhere new with a friend or family member.

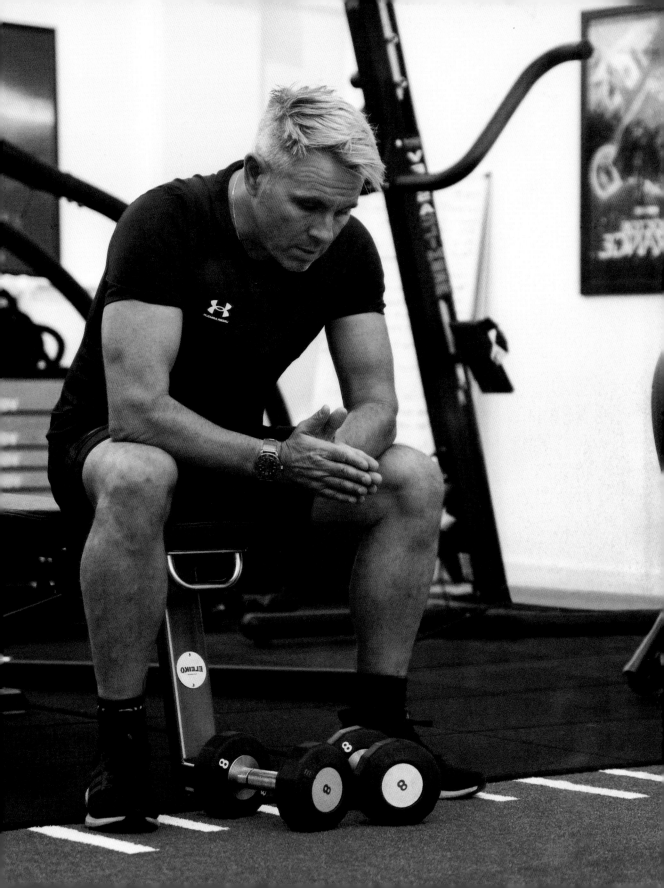

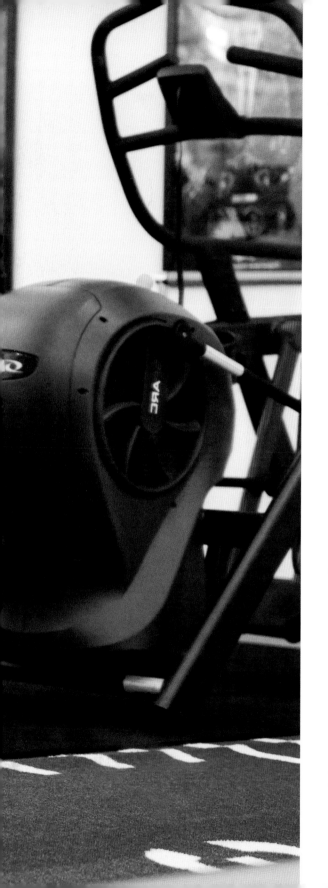

WEEK 10

'IT WAS A DREAM TO
WORK WITH SIMON.
HE PUSHED MY
BOUNDARIES AND
MADE ME WORK
HARD, BUT IT WAS SO
MUCH FUN.'
Léa Seydoux

THE SURPRISE THAT LETS YOU FEEL THE RESULTS

I don't think many other trainers would dare do this, but right at the end of this programme, when you might be expecting the intensity to be at its highest, I'm going to take you all the way back to Week 1.

ACCUMULATOR: 5–2

In this final week of the programme, I'm going to be asking you to go back to the start, and to do the exact same workouts that you did right at the beginning of this process. Psychologically, this is really important as it allows you to see how far you've progressed, physically and mentally, during this challenge.

This might feel ridiculous, or just too easy after everything you've done over the past nine weeks.

But consider how difficult you found these workouts in the beginning. Maybe you felt a bit unsteady and gasped for breath as you worked your way through the initial exercises. Perhaps in Week 1 you did this workout and you had to lie down with your legs in the air, or you needed a nap on the sofa for half an hour afterwards. And now you're thinking to yourself, 'This is nothing,' and you're realizing how much you have achieved in a relatively short period of time. 'Wow, I've accomplished so much,' is what you should be telling yourself. Be proud of the work you've done to change how you feel, look and move. Every time I've taken this approach with clients, rewinding all the way back to Week 1, they've loved the opportunity to prove to themselves how far they've come, because that's always going to make you feel amazing and give you a real sense of achievement.

FEEL THE DIFFERENCE

If you've lost a bit of weight feel free to put on a rucksack or a weighted vest one day this week, so you can feel how your body has changed during the challenge. The stresses you were putting on your cardiovascular system in Week 1 are now alleviated. Maybe your breathing used to be laboured and heavy, but now your lighter body is so much more efficient. Take a moment to reflect: that's how you used to be, how you used to function, and look at where you are today with your improved energy and stamina. There will be a glow about you that people will notice, especially if you haven't seen them since starting this programme.

YOUR REWARD

Feeling fit and mentally resilient is always going to be the greatest reward. But to mark getting to the end of this challenge, you might want to give yourself an additional reward with a new item of

WEEK 10 KIT LIST

BAND
BAR AND WEIGHTS
BENCH
BOX
DUMBBELLS
KETTLEBELL, PLATE
OR DUMBBELL
ROLLER

clothing. Every time you wear your new T-shirt, jeans or whatever else you buy, it will be a reminder of how successful you've been, and how many new habits you've created. Perhaps you need a whole new wardrobe. Your body composition has changed, giving you a chance to throw out some of your old clothes and refresh your style.

You're at the end of the ten weeks and the sense of achievement should be enormous. Enjoy that feeling. Although, of course, your fitness journey doesn't stop here …

YOU SHOULD BE PROUD OF YOURSELF. HAVE A MOMENT TO TAKE IN EVERYTHING YOU'VE ACCOMPLISHED OVER THE PAST NINE WEEKS.

WEEK 10 RECAP

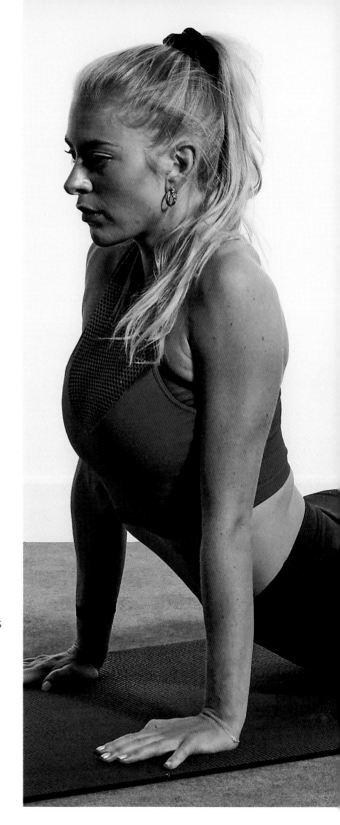

NUTRITION

O While an espresso is going to stimulate you, and you'll feel as though you have energy, remember that it contains hardly any calories. The body still has to find energy from somewhere and it's a good idea to eat post workout.

O Think about quality as well as quantity. Where possible, buy local and organic produce.

O Fruit, nuts and seeds are healthy, tasty snacks to have between meals.

WELLBEING

O Don't wait until you're tired before going to bed. Get into bed half an hour before you think you'll be tired. That could help you to have the best night's sleep.

O Keep a sleep diary. You might find that you can only sleep with a fuller stomach, which means eating a little later in the evening. See what works for you, including the environment within your bedroom, such as the lighting and the temperature.

O Look into whether you're sleeping on the right mattress for your body type and also whether you have the best pillow for your neck, shoulders and back.

O If you're able to, I can recommend having what I like to call an athlete's nap for up to twenty minutes during the day, which will help you to reboot and recharge.

ACCUMULATOR: 5–2

LEGS MONDAY	1: Squat 2: Band matrix 3: Lunge 4: Box step 5: Hip thrust
UPPER-BODY TUESDAY	1: Push-up 2: Shoulder matrix 3: Arms matrix 4: Barbell row 5: Clean and press
DYNAMICS WEDNESDAY	1: Bear crawl into pigeon 2: Bear crawl into cobra 3: Sit-up with lumbar twist 4: Side crab 5: Plyometric with a jump
CORE THURSDAY	1: Plank to pike to shoulder taps 2: Crunches, leg raises and heel taps 3: Abdominal rollout with a roller 4: Side obliques bend 5: Opposite elbow to knee crunch
FULL-BODY FRIDAY	1: Your weakest legs exercise 2: Push-up 3: Band matrix 4: Barbell row 5: Clean and press
ACTIVE SATURDAY	Take the chance to reconnect with a friend or family member. Perhaps you used to play tennis with them or run together.

WHAT NOW?

You've got through the ten weeks, and if you've closely followed my programme and my advice, I would hope that you've emerged fitter, stronger and mentally rejuvenated. But this isn't the time to ditch everything and just go back to what you were doing before you picked up this book. You've given yourself a foundation. Now the fresh challenge is to see whether you can lead more of an active life using the skills I've taught you. If this was all new to you, you've done the hardest part, which was getting started, but now you must try to keep your habits going and to make this part of your daily life. I hope I've given you the ability to enhance your physical and mental wellbeing for the long term, not just for ten weeks.

You've gone through short-term pain and had a medium-term goal (completing the challenge), but in the long term it's not so much about heading towards a destination as making fitness part of your lifestyle.

I appreciate that it's easy to get out of the habit of training, recovery and thinking about your nutrition, which is why it's important that you don't immediately let everything slide. Keep the good habits going, even if you don't necessarily have to train at quite the same intensity as you did during the challenge. Perhaps there will be elements of this programme that you can continue with indefinitely, and maybe with other parts you might feel as though dropping the intensity by 10 or 20 per cent will make it more sustainable for the long term.

My wish is that you use this book repeatedly for reference and motivation. This challenge isn't supposed to be something you do just once and then never again. By using the different rep levels and increasing the intensity, you can come back to this programme again as your fitness increases. And by adding some variety, such as mixing up what you do for cardio, and incorporating the additional core exercises that I shared with you, you can make it feel fresh the second or even third time. You might want to omit Week 10 when you revisit the programme, as that surprise won't have the same impact after the first time. One option could be to pick the weeks you think will give you the greatest benefit. You might, for instance, like to repeat Weeks 7, 8 and 9, being the most intense parts of the programme. But as I wrote in the introduction, you will get the most benefit from my programme if you follow the weeks chronologically, and you don't jump around and mix up the order.

Whatever you do, don't let your fitness drift. Now you've got momentum, how are you going to maintain that? Keep on challenging yourself!

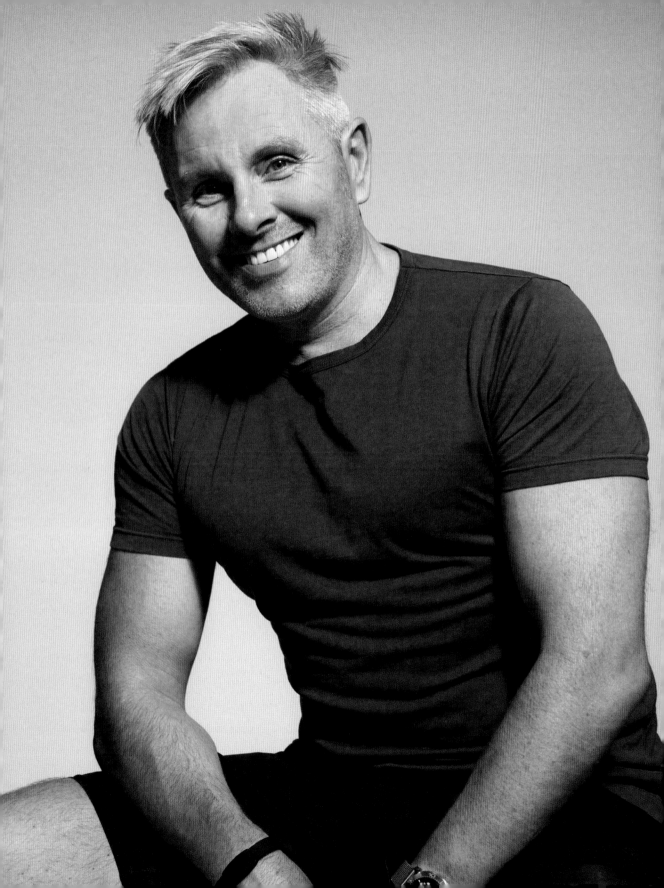

ACKNOWLEDGEMENTS

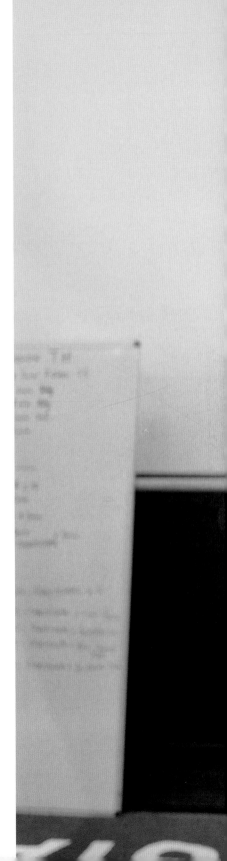

Tom Hiddleston's commitment to his health and fitness is inspiring to see. I'd also like to thank him for his kind words in the foreword.

I'm grateful to my other clients, in particular those who have provided quotes at the start of the chapters of this book. Greg Williams and his team went above and beyond to shoot the photography. I'm also indebted to Rich Peterson and Georgie Spurling for being the step-by-step models for this book. Rich is my right-hand man and always has my back, and Georgie is an inspirational health coach. For their constant support, I want to thank Jo Stansall and her team at Michael O'Mara, Nick Walters at David Luxton Associates and Mark Hodgkinson (even though he didn't bring as many biscuits to our writing sessions as he did for *Intelligent Fitness*).

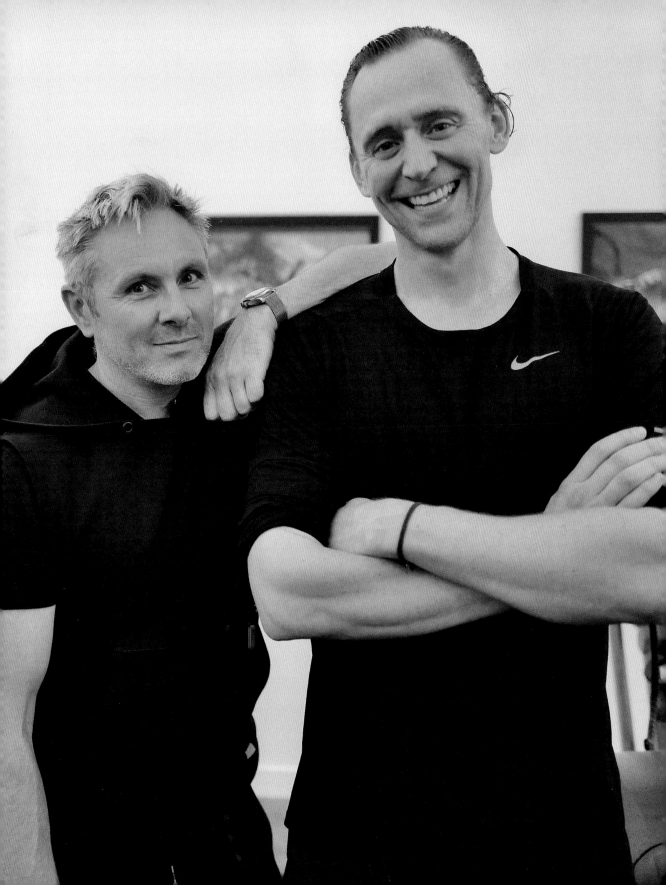

INDEX

V

W